C000084709

THE STACKING PLAN

*Stack on the good habits, lose the
bad ones, feel the benefits*

Sally Beare, dip BCNH, CNHC

Published by
Peach Publishing

To my beloved children, Araminta and Kublai

The Stacking Plan

What is The Stacking Plan?

The Stacking Plan is a ten-week plan in which each week you add just ONE healthy habit to your existing daily routine. For the rest of the day, every day that week, you carry on as usual. So, during the first week – Breakfast Week – you eat breakfast but carry on as normal for the rest of the day. During the second week – Fruit Week – you add fruit and you also carry on eating breakfast, and so on.

The idea is to 'stack' the good habits on top of each other until, at the end of the ten weeks, you are doing pretty much everything a person needs to be doing to eat a really good basic diet. This, along with some key lifestyle factors, should help you to enjoy optimum health as well as losing excess weight without having to diet.

The Stacking Plan is designed to make improving your eating habits as easy and enjoyable as possible, as well as being sustainable in the long term. You should find that most of the 'naughty' habits move to the background or even get squeezed out completely without your giving them much thought as you will be so busy eating all the right things. And if you do deviate, it doesn't matter – at least you know where you are supposed to be and how to get back there. Another aim of the Plan is to educate you in manageable, bite-sized pieces so you know *why* each habit can be of so much benefit to you.

The Stacking Plan is not a fad diet and it is not particularly complicated. Its basic essence is that it teaches you to incorporate everything your body needs in order to be in good health, at the same time as giving you the information you need to make the right choices for you. The Plan embraces the idea of eating all kinds of different foods, and it includes wisdom from Paleolithic eating, traditional diets, raw food diets and other diets without being too limiting. This means that you are likely to find plenty to eat that you really enjoy and should not 'fall off the wagon' since there is not really a 'wagon' to fall off.

Huge numbers of people have real problems today in terms of health, and one of the main reasons for this is what we are eating. Many of us eat food, or 'food', which has deviated far from what we are naturally supposed to eat, and our bodies do not function well as a result. I am certain that if everybody ate foods and did things which were good for them, this would be of immeasurable benefit not just to each of us but to entire populations, nations, our descendants, and in fact, not to sound too grandiose or anything, the entire planet.

How The Stacking Plan Can Help You

The aim of The Stacking Plan is to help you to feel and look better, stay younger for longer, avoid chronic disease, and shed unwanted weight, *for good*, all by eating food that tastes good and by doing things you enjoy.

The Plan helps you to stack on the good habits one by one, and slowly wean yourself off bad habits without having to go 'cold turkey' or feel deprived. For some this may be a slight change, for others it may be a major overhaul. Either way, it is designed to be as easy and as enjoyable as possible. With The Stacking Plan, you can also learn, in easy steps, about what is good for your physical and mental health, and why, and what will do you harm, and why.

The aim of The Stacking Plan is not to enable weight loss *per se*. However, being at the right weight for you is integral to good health. When people start to eat the things which feed their bodies in the right way, they almost always start to lose excess weight, or to put it on if they are underweight. Many diets cause temporary weight loss, but with the side-effect of missing out on nutrients, which can cause problems. The Stacking Plan is the other way around because it enables you to get the right nutrients whilst having the beneficial side-effect of aiding weight loss where it is needed.

Where did The Stacking Plan come from?

The Stacking Plan is the product of a happy union between modern nutrition science and ancient wisdom. The 'modern nutrition science' part comes from the latest scientific research from nutrition experts as well as my training and clinical practice as a nutritional therapist. The 'ancient wisdom' part comes from my research into some remarkable places in the world which I call the 'Longevity Hot Spots', which I have written about in my previous books. In these places, disease levels are exceptionally low and people frequently live very long lives without suffering from illness. You can read more about the Longevity Hot Spots in my books, *50 Secrets of the World's Longest-Living People* (Avalon, US, 2006) and *The Live-Longer Diet* (Piatkus, UK, 2003) (also published as *The Anti-Ageing Diet*).

I have included some recipes whose principles are based on nutrition science, my own trial-and-error creations and real-life recipes beloved of the people who live in the Longevity Hot Spots. Once you know the principles of healthful eating, it is easy to find endless more recipes on the internet or to create your own – mine are just a starting point.

Losing weight with The Stacking Plan

Dieting tends to make people fatter, for various reasons. One is that not being allowed certain things, as with everything in life, makes us want those things even more. Another is that dieting makes us hungry, and in the end we give in and eat – often retrospectively ('I wasn't allowed chocolate brownies when I was on my diet so I'm going to have three now to make up for it'). Thirdly, during a period of food deprivation, it is thought that the body compensates for what it thinks is a food shortage by slowing the metabolism down and storing any calories it can as fat so that the dieter can survive long enough to reproduce.

Studies also show that people tend to feel hungrier than ever and to gain weight after going on a diet (1). This is most likely because of the 'hunger hormone', ghrelin. In a study of dieters, overweight men and women were put on a strict diet. At the end of the diet they were encouraged to start eating healthfully. Initially, they lost a significant amount of weight. However, ultimately they put on weight readily and were hungrier than before they started dieting. The researchers found that levels of ghrelin were up by 20 per cent, making the subjects feel hungry. Additionally, levels of peptide YY, the hormone which switches off appetite, were lower (2).

Doing The Stacking Plan means you can rule out dieting, calorie counting, and fretting on the scales. You will simply be eating, and doing, what you need to keep you at the right weight for you. You can eat plenty of food and not go hungry. Cravings should disappear, and your metabolism should improve. By taking regular exercise and reducing stress levels you can also balance your insulin and cortisol levels, which can help to reduce excess weight. Remember: *slow and steady wins the race*. You want to be a tortoise, not a hare, for effective weight loss, even if you do look like a gazelle by the end of it.

The Stacking Plan and Paleo eating

If you have tried Paleolithic (or 'hunter-gatherer') eating, you may have found it very helpful for health and weight loss. In his book, *The Paleo Diet*, Paleo expert Dr Loren Cordain explains how our diet no longer suits our biochemistry. For millions of years, we ate what we could catch, pick, or gather; namely meat, seafood, fruit, and vegetables, and it is only very recently in human history that we have started eating other foods, such as wheat, cheese, and sugar, which are very convenient, but are not part of our natural diet.

The Paleo theory makes perfect sense in many ways. However, I personally and most others I come across find it very difficult, if not impossible, to follow a strict Paleo diet. For vegetarians it poses obvious problems, whilst others, such as myself, just don't like eating a lot of meat and seafood, not least because it is tricky on a household budget to eat organic, free-range, grass-fed meat or wild fish at every meal. Pieces of cold meat or fish don't work for my children in school lunchboxes – they would actually rather starve - and I just can't pledge never to eat a flapjack, or Parmesan cheese for that matter, again.

In the Longevity Hot Spots I have studied and in other places renowned for the excellent health of their inhabitants, the diet is not a Paleo one. Grains and legumes are eaten, and although you would have to take the exact same populations and feed them a Paleo diet in order to discover whether they fared even better on the Paleo one, the fact is that these populations have excellent health records with very low levels of chronic disease. In Nicoya in Costa Rica, for example, where an unusually high number of ninety-plus-year-olds can be found bounding around without a health care in the world, people eat beans and rice almost three times a day.

So, with The Stacking Plan, I have taken a bit of a middle ground. If you wish to do The Stacking Plan and also follow a Paleo diet, that is perfectly possible – you just have to make sure to choose certain protein foods and avoid certain carbohydrates, using the information given in Proteins Week and Carbohydrates Week. Equally, if you are a vegetarian or vegan, you can use the information in Weeks Four and Five to make your choices carefully. It must be remembered that the point of this book is to set you on the right path in terms of basic eating habits – having got that in place you can then finesse your way of eating further if you want to.

The Stacking Plan and 5:2 fasting

If you have been doing a diet where you 'fast', or restrict calories, on certain days during the week, such as one of the '5:2' diet plans, and you find it effective for you, you should find that you can carry on doing so easily with The Stacking Plan. The Plan will help you learn how to eat foods which are good for you on the non-fasting days of the week too, which will enhance the benefits of eating the 5:2 way. For more about the 5:2 way of eating, see Digestion Week.

Why modern medicine cannot save us

Modern medicine has its place and of course it saves lives. Serious accidents, difficult childbirth, life-threatening infectious diseases – modern medicine can prevent all of these and more from taking our lives.

However, modern medicine cannot do anything to prevent the onset of killer chronic diseases such as heart disease and cancer, or to slow their rising incidence, and it does not enable the body to heal itself. Nor is it able to slow the ageing process: researchers have found that in countries such as the US and the UK, we are now ageing a huge *fifteen years* faster than older generations and developing medical problems which are worse than those of our forebears, despite all the miracles of modern medicine (3). Where the number one killers are concerned, modern medicine is a patch-up job at best, and most of the time it's too little, too late.

Pharmaceutical drugs can extend lifespan and reduce pain. However, they do not resolve the root cause of chronic disease, and they are often dangerous. Of the 98,000 - 250,000 deaths caused by medical mishap annually in the USA the vast majority are due to pharmaceutical drugs (4, 5), and there is a similar pattern in the UK.

Statins, to take an example of one commonly-used drug which is taken by millions of people in the US and the UK, have been associated with cognitive impairment, liver dysfunction, renal failure, and diabetes (6). We also know that the pharmaceuticals industry has a habit of 'disease-mongering' - inventing illnesses which will require a pill to 'fix' them (7). Prevention is better than cure, especially when the 'cure' can be fatal.

Eating and doing the right things means that you can take your health into your own hands, so that fate and the pharmaceuticals industry don't have all the power. One recent study of over 23,000 German adults, for example, showed those who did not smoke, had a good diet, were not overweight, and took exercise had ninety three per cent less diabetes, eighty one per cent lower heart disease, fifty per cent less stroke, and thirty six per cent less cancer than others (8). And, according to Rachael Stolzenberg-Solomon, a researcher at the National

Cancer Institute, 'The easiest and least expensive way to reduce your risk for cancer is just by eating a healthy diet'(9).

Knowing this and learning what we need to eat and do to stay healthy makes the idea of illness much less frightening. We can all have a lot more control over our health than we currently do, and one of the main aims of The Stacking Plan is to help you to take that control.

The Stacking Plan and specific illness

Eating the right way can have a dramatic effect on a wide range of health conditions, without necessarily having to find a 'magic bullet'. Unexplained tiredness, random aches and pains, headaches, indigestion and other complaints are likely to clear up when the diet is cleaned up, even if their exact cause is unknown. That is because what is good for one part of your body is likely to be good for the rest of it. In the words of the great physician Hippocrates himself, 'all disease begins in the gut.'

There is, therefore, up to a point, a basic 'one diet fits all' principle, in that the vast majority of us need roughly the same things. We need the right proteins, the right carbs, the right fats, and so on, in the right amounts and the right ratios. The Stacking Plan aims to address that. Generally, in my practice, no matter what the illness of the client I am seeing, there will be some basic eating principles the client needs to follow in order to address their health problems.

Nutritional therapy, however, can also address specific illnesses with specific diets. For example, if somebody has kidney stones or low immunity or gout or inflammatory bowel disease, to take just a few examples of many, they will need to tailor their diet accordingly and may also need particular supplements. Also, some people can digest certain foods better than others, either because of existing health conditions or because of their genetic predisposition.

This means that although The Stacking Plan can educate

you as to what is a basic optimum diet, it is beyond the scope of this book to address specific health conditions requiring specific treatment. So, if you have health issues which do not clear up of their own accord by eating well, and you wish to follow the nutrition route, I recommend that you see a well-qualified, expert nutritional therapist in order to make the best use of specific nutrients or to cut out certain foods – you can, of course, do this in tandem with The Stacking Plan. If you are on medication, always check with your doctor before taking supplements, and it might also be a good idea to discuss your healthful eating changes with them.

Why and How The Stacking Plan Works

For millions of years, we humans and our pre-human ancestors ate nothing other than what you might call 'real' food. Now, all of a sudden, we aren't doing that any more. Where once we could only eat things we could catch or pick, such as fish, berries, and leaves, today we are able to incorporate large amounts of manufactured 'foods' such as crisps, white bread, and processed cheese.

Our bodies do not do well on this recent new diet, because it does not contain the right types and amounts of proteins, carbohydrates and fibre (macronutrients) or vitamins and minerals (micronutrients) they need. This means that our bodies simply cannot function optimally and become vulnerable to all kinds of disease.

For example, our brains need B vitamins and essential fatty acids; our adrenal glands need vitamin C and magnesium; our guts need probiotics and vitamin A; our bones need calcium, magnesium and vitamin D, and so on. Without these nutrients it is only a matter of time before we run into problems.

We are also doing things which actively damage our health. Processed and refined foods, a sedentary lifestyle, and stress all work together to create disease-making conditions for our bodies. It takes a bit of effort not to eat and live this way, because of the way modern living and eating works, and so it has become the norm for most people. Smoking was once common-place in developed countries, and people did it because everyone else did it, it was addictive, and nobody realised how lethal it was. Now it's just the same, but with the modern diet.

The result is widespread chronic illness which undermines quality of life, especially after a certain age. It is now estimated that seventy five per cent of diseases in Western countries such as the US and the UK are preventable illnesses caused by a poor diet and lifestyle (1). Heart disease, cancer, obesity and diabetes are some of the biggest killers, and they are all strongly diet-related.

In the 'Longevity Hot Spots' I have studied, rates of these illnesses are at the lowest levels anywhere in the world, and people there have the highest life expectancy levels on the planet (2). When people do die, it is not unusual for them to die quietly in their sleep without having ever suffered a day's illness. The reason for this is mainly to do with what they are eating and doing. It has less to do with genes than habits, we know, because when these people migrate to other places they start to get the same diseases as the native inhabitants there (3).

By doing The Stacking Plan you should be able to do all the right things nutritionally and incorporate the lifestyle habits which go hand-in-hand with good eating to create vibrant health. The result is that you can slow your rate of ageing and significantly reduce your chances of suffering from chronic disease. You should also find that minor aches and pains, mood swings, hormonal imbalances and cravings lessen or vanish. At the same time, you will become knowledgeable about what you need to do and why. This means that to a large extent you can take your health into your own hands.

Another potentially dramatic effect of The Stacking Plan is that you can help your children and, believe it or not, even your children's children to have better health. Scientists now know that what we eat affects not just our DNA, but that of our descendants. We are what our grandparents ate, and our grandchildren will be what we eat. So, even if not for us, it seems foolish not to keep ourselves well for future generations.

Five ways in which The Stacking Plan can keep you younger for longer

Here are some of the key ways in which The Stacking Plan can help slow the ageing process and significantly reduce your risk of getting chronic diseases such as cancer and heart disease:

1. It helps balance blood sugar and insulin levels

If you want to age quickly and suffer from illness, have a blood sugar imbalance (most of us do). If you want to age slowly and be well, start by balancing your blood sugar levels. That's how powerful the effect of sugar, or glucose, is. If you experience sugar cravings, irritability when you miss a meal, and energy slumps during the day, you almost certainly have a blood sugar imbalance. Nearly every one of us eating a modern diet does to some extent, but it's never too late to change, and this is one of the most important things which The Stacking Plan addresses.

Whenever you eat a pastry, white bread, cake, or sugar, or when you feel stressed, your blood sugar levels spike and your insulin rushes out to try and tether the glucose away in cells to use for energy and to stop it from damaging blood vessels, as it does. Insulin, being an ancient hormone in a modern world, is trying its best to do its job, but it struggles to cope. When we eat sugar, too much insulin is released, blood glucose levels drop too low, we crave sugar in order to get them back up again, and so the vicious cycle continues.

Most of us have both blood sugar and blood insulin swings, and both cause accelerated ageing to blood vessels and cells. The problem is made worse as we age because our cells develop 'insulin resistance' after years of this abuse and this means more insulin and glucose circulating round the blood vessels trying to get into our cells.

The ultimate result can be excess weight, damage (including wrinkles) from a process called 'glycosylation', adult-onset diabetes, heart disease, and cancer, all of which are linked with excess insulin. Excess insulin is also connected with shorter telomeres, stretches of DNA on our chromosomes whose length is strongly connected with the rate at which we age (4).

The Stacking Plan is designed to help balance blood sugar and insulin levels in a multi-pronged approach. The foods eaten are low on the Glycaemic Index (a marker of how much glucose is released by certain foods) and contain the right kinds and amounts of protein, carbohydrates and fats. Low stress and regular exercise are also key factors in balancing blood sugar and insulin levels.

2. It provides antioxidant power

As we age, wear and tear accumulates in our cells and DNA, largely due to free radicals, rogue molecules which rampage through our bodies damaging other molecules by 'oxidising' them. If you watch an apple going brown, that is because it is oxidising. A similar process happens to our bodies over time. It is as though we are slowly cooking.

We have our own antioxidant systems but it is not enough to neutralise the damage caused by the high amounts of free radicals which bombard us every day from pollution, the wrong food, toxins, and other sources; our bodies are also designed to take in large amounts of antioxidants from food which these days most of us do not do.

By making sure we get plenty of antioxidant-rich foods in our diet we can protect ourselves from free radical damage. Plant foods are high in antioxidants, because they need them to protect themselves from ageing, so when we eat high-antioxidant plant foods, such as fruit and vegetables, we get those benefits too. The Stacking Plan minimises sources of damaging free radicals and is high in antioxidants from a variety of food sources.

3. It is anti-inflammatory

Too much inflammation in the body, a common situation today, is closely linked with accelerated ageing and chronic diseases such as heart disease and cancer, so in order to stay healthier for longer we need to keep inflammation levels down (5). You can think of chronic inflammation as being in a permanently overheated state, with little fires burning all around your body.

The Stacking Plan helps put out those 'fires' since it provides plenty of anti-inflammatory plant foods and anti-inflammatory fats and restricts pro-inflammatory foods such as sugar, alcohol and unhealthy fats. Avoiding stress and taking regular exercise are also effective ways to reduce chronic inflammation.

Excess inflammation is closely linked with the other four major factors in ageing discussed here - blood sugar swings, free radicals, cortisol and the immune system, so you can see how the jigsaw fits together. What is wonderful about eating the right foods is that it addresses all of these together, and you don't have to worry about understanding the science. It just works.

4. It keeps cortisol levels down

Levels of the stress hormone, cortisol, increase with age as wear and tear accumulates in the part of the brain which regulates cortisol use. Cortisol itself is ageing, because it is toxic to certain brain cells, it blocks anti-inflammatory prostaglandins, it damages the thymus and hence the immune system, it causes weight gain, it accelerates bone loss and it shortens telomeres. The life cycle of the Pacific salmon is a good illustration of the damaging effects of cortisol: after reproducing, the poor salmon, for whom evolution has no further use, is flooded with cortisol and dies a sudden death.

The Stacking Plan keeps cortisol levels down by keeping blood sugar levels steady and helping prevent inflammation which leads to cortisol release. Low stress and regular exercise are also cortisol-lowering factors in the Plan.

5. It keeps the immune system strong

Our immune systems decline with age, making us more susceptible to illness and chronic inflammation. The thymus, a crucial part of the immune system, atrophies (shrivels) so that less immune T-cells are produced, auto-immunity can become over-zealous leading to autoimmune conditions such as rheumatoid arthritis, and our immune bodies have less ability to destroy pathogens and cancer cells.

The Stacking Plan helps keep the immune system strong even as we age by providing antioxidants, vitamins and minerals, the right amount of protein, and essential fatty acids. Substances which stress the immune system such as sugar, free radical-producing foods, and excess caffeine and alcohol are minimised. Exercise, low stress, and plenty of sleep also all help to keep the immune system strong.

The Stacking Plan can help you look younger too

So that's what is going on inside your body. But what about on the outside? Doing The Stacking Plan can help your outside reflect what is going on inside. To start with, it can help give you younger-looking skin. The antioxidants in all the fruit and vegetables protect skin cells from aging free-radical damage, whilst antioxidant carotenoids are thought to give a healthy glow to skin (6). Beneficial fats keep skin cells plump and elastic, and hydrating drinks help keep toxins out and skin clear. Avoiding sugar and refined carbohydrates helps get rid of acne.

Getting plenty of nutrients is also good for hair condition, since hair reflects intake of minerals, proteins, and the right fats. Nails will benefit from the mineral intake, and eyes should become clearer. And, most welcome of all to some, doing the Stacking Plan means eating and doing all the right things to boost metabolism and shift stubborn excess weight.

Do you have any of the following symptoms?

These are just some of the symptoms that can improve with the Stacking Plan.

- Low or fluctuating energy levels
- Excess weight
- Food cravings
- Mood swings or depression
- Poor skin, nail and hair condition
- Headaches
- Constipation
- Poor digestion
- Frequent coughs and colds
- Allergies
- Low immunity
- Insomnia
- Unidentified aches and pains
- High blood pressure
- High cholesterol levels
- Blood sugar imbalance, syndrome X or diabetes Type II
- Inflammatory conditions
- Premenstrual stress

What People Have Said About The Stacking Plan

'I love The Stacking Plan as it gives you control over your food, not the other way round like with usual diet plans. This way I'm the boss, not my eating habits, which has always scuppered my success in losing weight in the past.'
Claire

'I have really enjoyed and benefited massively from the Plan and all your advice – thank you! And I have lost almost a stone since I last weighed myself before doing the Plan.'
Ollie

'Doing the Stacking Plan has been such a revelation . . . it's been life-changing. I'm really really pleased I did it.'
Jason

'There aren't any other books which actually teach you how to eat.'
Claudia

'Your diet hasn't just given me a fish, it has taught me *how* to fish.'
Natasha

'I feel SO much better. Why has it taken me so long to do this?'
Grace

'I have been getting frequent compliments on how well, young, and radiant I am looking. I've twice been asked if I am in love, and I've even been told that I really don't look any older than I did 20 years ago! Now at last, I feel I'm coming to the end of the search for my perfect diet.'
Clare

'Since starting the Plan three weeks ago I've lost half a stone – and I haven't once felt that I had to 'diet' or go hungry.'
Misha

'I'm feeling amazing – light and free! I have released 3lbs since I started this way of eating. I'm super-happy about this! I'm ready for my body to reflect how wonderful I feel physically and mentally on the inside.'
Joanne

'I found out this week that making good choices is easy because I read your instructions every morning and prepare mentally. This week I experienced better elimination; realized that I am not sleepy after dinner and I never get tired.'
Beverly

'Has it been six weeks already? Love the way this change in eating is helping me feel better with more long-lasting energy and the change in my skin and complexion is even getting comments from people around me.'
Johnna

'I am shocked at how differently my body is responding to my new eating habits. We went out to dinner last night and I was so conscious of what was on my plate and how much to eat of each. No more cravings.'
Vicki

'The photo attached shows me in a suit that I have not been able to wear in more than a year. Whoop whoop!'
Amy

'My husband looked at me after he finished his meal and said, 'that was awesome! I don't feel gross or bloated or like I need to lie down for a nap at all.'
Amy

'Thanks to The Stacking Plan I have finally been able to step

off the daily blood sugar rollercoaster and return to the ideal weight of my youth. The discovery of delicious new foods and ways of eating has made it so easy.'
Simon

'I have noticed myself being full quicker and my energy levels are higher. I have also noticed this week more regular bowel elimination. Also, my kids who are 12 and 16 have been influenced by my healthier eating and preparation of food. I have also lost three pounds!'
Becky

'Increasing my servings of vegetables wasn't as hard as I thought. I used not to like many cooked vegetables, but there are so many different, tasty ways to fix them that I've become a fan of many.'
Debbie

'My skin seems to be clearing up. Normally when I have my period, my skin breaks out, but this week it was remarkably calm.'
Leonie

'This is the longest I have managed to stay on an eating programme – I am so proud of myself.'

Purnima

The Stacking Plan

How to use the Plan

The Stacking Plan is a simple-to-use ten-week plan. It is NOT a plan in which you have to eat nothing but celery and sprouted chick peas, avoid all your favourite foods, and count the minutes until the ten weeks are up. That would simply not be enjoyable or sustainable.

What it means, just to recap, is that each week, you add ONE good new habit to your existing dietary routine. You can carry on doing everything else just as you were already. For example, if all you eat is steak pies, the first week, you can carry on doing so, but you add a nutrient-rich breakfast in as well. The next week, you continue eating steak pies if you wish, but the breakfasts stay and you also add a piece or two of daily fruit, and so on. This is why it's called 'The Stacking Plan', because each week you 'stack on' a new good habit.

By the end of the ten-week plan you should be well on your way to eating and doing all the right things, without having felt that you have had to go on a diet or make a sudden and radical overhaul of your existing habits. You should also be very well-armed with information about what is good for your body and why.

If you have a lot of not-so-healthy habits, try not to worry about those just now or to feel intimidated about giving them up. The aim of the Plan is to help you to gradually squeeze out those habits almost without thinking about it, by taking on good habits instead. And if you already eat well, you may not be doing anything dramatic by following The Stacking Plan - it may just involve a little tweaking of what you already do.

Of course, if you wish to, you can read through to the end straight away and do the whole ten 'weeks' at once. You can also make each 'week' last for as long as you like, although I recommend trying to keep it to a week (perhaps two at the most), so as to keep the momentum going. You may also find that you need to take a break from the plan for a few days due to, for example, social functions or holidays. If you do that, simply carry on from where you left off as soon as you can. As time goes on, your new good habits should start to become ingrained, so that you don't have to think too hard about what you are doing. It will just feel right.

Ideally, you will end up eating and doing things which are good for you, if not all of the time, then *most of the time* and, very importantly, *enjoying doing so*. In the long term, this means that even if guilty pleasures such as cake, chocolate, or crisps, for example, find their way into your life from time to time, you should be able to take them or leave them without feeling that they have power over you. If you are someone who is always trying to give these things up and regularly over-indulging in them, you should find that, if you do the right things most of the time, you don't feel so bad about having 'treats' sometimes, and you are likely to find that you want them less anyway.

There are some important lifestyle habits which go hand-in-hand with good eating habits, such as taking regular exercise and reducing stress. You can read about those in the section called *The Stacking Plan: What to Do*. You can read this section at any point whilst you are doing The Stacking Plan, but the sooner the better. You should find that these lifestyle habits greatly enhance everything else you are doing.

Meet my 'human guinea pigs'

During the course of the ten weeks, you can follow the progress of my 'human guinea pigs', Claire and Ollie. I think it is fair to say that both Claire and Ollie were eating badly and feeling bad at the start of the Plan, and that both were eating well and feeling well by the end. It was wonderful to witness this transformation, and the ease with which they made it, and I hope that readers will experience something similar. You can read about their progress at the end of each chapter.

Claire, 43, wanted to sort out her immune system, as she had a lingering chest infection, and to lose some weight, ideally around two stone. She also tended to get constipated and suffered from haemorrhoids as well as possible IBS. She was worried about bowel and colon cancer, and she had also recently been diagnosed with a heart murmur. She wanted to be eating well, but found it hard. 'To be honest, I'm an emotional eater, and it's the night time for me that's the problem as that's the time I'm most likely to eat rubbish', she said. 'I really want to sort my days out so my nights aren't spent snacking on rubbish. If I don't sort it out now, my health is going to be a major issue for me. I know my life is in my own hands.'

Ollie, 35, takes plenty of exercise and is of course still young, but at the time of starting The Stacking Plan he was overweight, and he had high cholesterol which he was concerned about as it runs in his family. He also had regular sugar cravings and corresponding energy highs and lows, and he was eating a lot of convenience foods. He knew these weren't doing him any good but, as he said, 'my willpower is not great.' Ollie wanted to make changes, but he didn't know how to do it.

And now, the Plan begins. I recommend that you choose a day to start, preferably today or tomorrow if you can, find a quiet half hour to read the information, and go. Try to start each week on the same day so that you don't let the days slip by without moving onto the following week. Don't delay starting because you think you might have to give something up this week – you don't!

1

Breakfast Week

People often tell me they miss breakfast because they don't feel very hungry first thing in the morning, and skipping breakfast makes them feel quite pleased with themselves, as though they are successfully dieting and don't really need food.

But then mid-morning comes, and they are starving and lose control over the biscuits or flapjacks, perhaps washing it all down with a large cappuccino for good measure. This creates a blood sugar yo-yo effect with first too little blood sugar and then too much, leading to energy highs and lows and cravings carrying on throughout the day. This often culminates in a large supper, which doesn't really get digested properly during the night, especially as it can often be wolfed down with minimal chewing, and so the person in question isn't really hungry again next morning and the whole cycle starts again.

This scenario is very common, with many people missing breakfast, even though it is probably the most important meal of the day. Between ten and fifteen per cent of adults don't eat a morning meal, whilst a 2010 study showed that around one third of school pupils usually go without (1).

Missing breakfast is more likely to make you fat than slim, since blood sugar swings ultimately cause weight gain because of the effect they have on insulin and the storage of glucose as fat, as well as causing irresistible cravings for sweet (fattening) foods. Also, our circadian rhythms work in such a way that we burn calories from breakfast more efficiently than those eaten later in the day. Several studies show, in fact, that those who miss breakfast are more likely to be overweight or obese than those who eat it (2, 3).

Missing breakfast has been shown in many studies to lead to accelerated ageing and chronic disease, largely due to its effect on blood sugar and insulin levels. A large-scale study published in the *American Journal of Clinical Nutrition* in 2012 showed that men who skip breakfast are more likely to get type 2 diabetes, cancer and heart disease than those who eat it, even after quality of diet is taken into account (4).

Dieting teenagers take note – eating breakfast not only helps keep you slim, it also leads to better mental performance, since the brain relies on a steady supply of glucose for its fuel. A study from the American Dietetic Association in 2005 found that children and adolescents who eat breakfast perform better when it comes to memory and test grades (5). That goes for adults too, of course.

When you eat breakfast, make sure you avoid eating a sugary breakfast, since this can disrupt blood sugar levels as much as avoiding breakfast can, by causing a blood sugar spike which will be followed by a blood sugar trough. It's easy to snatch a sweet breakfast when we are tired and in a rush in the mornings, but that gets our blood sugar levels off to a bad start and will only cause more tiredness later, as well as more sweet cravings. The best breakfasts for balancing blood sugar contain some form of protein and good fats (see the Proteins and Fats weeks for more on these – for now, proteins and good fats are included in the breakfast ideas below).

If you are usually not hungry at breakfast time, try having a smaller supper the night before, which should leave you hungrier in the morning (as well as being better for your digestion). If you find you need an hour or so before your appetite wakes up, try to arrange your schedule so that you can have breakfast once you return from the school run or arrive at the office or get back from the gym, or whatever it is you do first thing. But do make sure you eat breakfast before you reach a state of mid-morning starvation and are ready to kill for a pastry.

Mid-morning snacks

If you find that, despite eating breakfast, you are very hungry mid-morning, have a snack to keep you going until lunch time, otherwise your blood sugar levels may sink too low. A good snack could be fruit (see Fruit Week for more on this subject), a nutrient-rich smoothie containing proteins and fats, a handful of nuts and seeds, or oat cakes with hummus or avocado. See also 'Snack Ideas' in the Recipes section.

Breakfast ideas

These breakfast recipes are aimed to give you lasting energy and a good dose of nutrients.

The cereal killer

Cereal is easy and convenient and it provides a quick fix, but in terms of health, the majority of mass-produced cereals are absolutely the wrong way to start the day. Most breakfast cereals are extremely high in sugar – in a UK study, 60 per cent of cereals were found to contain more sugar per serving than a jam doughnut, and many to contain more than a chocolate bar. Most cereals also contain roasted grains which are difficult to digest. What this means in terms of health is blood sugar and insulin swings, higher triglycerides and harmful LDL cholesterol, and more inflammation – all risk factors for cardiovascular disease, cancer and diabetes. If you must have cereal, choose low-sugar ones which contain nuts, seeds and fruit, or add your own to bump up the nutrient value.

Porridge Plus

Some people like porridge, some people don't, some people quite like it but find it isn't enough in the morning. Porridge is actually a useful and versatile breakfast dish to which you can make all kinds of flavour- and nutrient-enhancing additions to keep you fuller for longer.

<u>Ingredients (serves one)</u>

This porridge uses a range of grains and pseudograins which provide more protein and other nutrients than simple porridge oats, as well as flax seed for protein and good fats (I have referred to flax seed as 'ground flax seed', but you can also buy ground sprouted flax seed which is more digestible so use that if you can get it). As a result this is a more fulfilling porridge recipe which provides longer-lasting energy.

If you can, it is best to ferment these grains overnight before using them so as to reduce their content of anti-nutrients – there is more about this in the Proteins and Carbohydrate weeks and fermenting instructions in the Recipes section.

1 cup mixed whole oat flakes, buckwheat flakes, millet flakes, and/or quinoa flakes (available in good health food shops or from online suppliers) - you can use any combination of these
1 cup oat milk or soy milk (optional) and water as required
2 tablespoons live plain yoghurt or soy yoghurt
1-2 tablespoons ground flax seed
2 tablespoons nuts and/or seeds
Maple syrup or honey

Mix the porridge flakes in a pan with some water and the oat or soy milk (if you are using it) and stir over a moderate heat. Add more liquid as needed to give the porridge the texture you desire. When the porridge is cooked, stir in the ground flax seeds. Serve topped with yoghurt, fresh unsalted nuts and/ or seeds, and a trickle of maple syrup or honey if you feel the need for a little sweetener.

Savoury toast

Toast with jam or honey is not a great way to start the day because it lacks protein and is on the sugary side, so will get blood sugar levels off on the wrong foot. Toast and jam is also not very inspiring. Furthermore, wheat causes problems with digestion for many people (there is more on this in Carbohydrates Week).

Savoury toast is a better idea both in terms of interest and nutrient value. Try using pumpernickel bread, sprouted pumpernickel bread, essene bread or sourdough rye for your toast rather than wheat bread as they are more digestible and higher in nutrients. If you do eat wheat, make it whole wheat. Try drizzling olive oil over your toast, as they do in Mediterranean countries, rather than using butter or spreads.

Try some of the following:

- Toast with poached, boiled or scrambled eggs (see below for more about eggs)
- Toast with eggs, sautéed tomatoes, avocado, capers and herbs
- Toast with kippers
- Toast with sardines
- Baked beans on toast
- Toast with hummus or home-made bean dip
- Toast with sliced avocado or guacamole
- Toast with yeast spread
- Toast with nut butter (and all-fruit jam if you wish)

Wheat-free pancakes

You can make pancakes with ordinary wheat flour for now if you are certain you don't have a problem digesting wheat (again, see Carbohydrates Week for more on this); but make it whole wheat or at the very least, a mix of white flour and whole grain flour.

I make pancakes with a random blend of wheat-free flours, such as buckwheat, millet, quinoa, oat, amaranth or rye flour, depending on what I have at home. For a well-textured flexible pancake, it is best to add buckwheat and/or rye flour, otherwise the pancakes can come out a bit stiff.

If you happen to have porridge flakes made from any of the grains listed above, such as buckwheat or millet flakes, you can turn them into flour by putting them dry in the blender for a few seconds. Go for whole-grain, non-refined products.

As with porridge, you can ferment the grains you use in your pancake mixture to make them more digestible – see the Recipes section on how to do this.

Ingredients (serves 1-2)

1-2 cups any combination of buckwheat flour, rye flour, millet flour, quinoa flour, oat flour, amaranth flour
1-2 tablespoon ground flax seed
1 teaspoon baking powder
1-2 eggs (optional)
½ cup ground almonds (optional – adds flavour and protein)
2 cups oat milk (if oat milk is not available you can use soy milk or rice milk or yoghurt and water)
1 banana *or* the grated zest of one lemon (optional)
1 teaspoon vanilla
Water (if necessary, to thin the mixture)

Combine all the ingredients in a blender, adding enough liquid to make the mixture easy to pour – it should be not too thick, and not too thin.

To cook the pancake, use a non-stick pan or melt a small knob of coconut oil, ghee, or butter in a frying pan. Get the pan nice and hot (this stops the pancake from sticking) and pour in the mixture, thinning it out by tilting the pan. Cook until golden on both sides – about 2-3 minutes each side. You may need to make the pancakes fairly small so that they are easier to flip.

Try serving with nut butter and a little all-fruit jam, maple syrup, honey, lemon juice, cinnamon, or yoghurt with berries.

Eggs – boiled, poached or scrambled

Eggs are a source of quality protein and make a good start to the day, especially where blood sugar levels are concerned. Some doctors' advice that eggs raise cholesterol levels is outdated and incorrect - for most, an egg a day will not pose a problem. Eggs can cause constipation, however, so if they have that effect on you, avoid having them too often.

Try always to use free-range organic eggs from grass-fed hens, since these are higher in nutrients and richer in flavour than ordinary eggs and also contain better levels of valuable omega 3 essential fats (you can read more about those in Fats Week). Poached, boiled and scrambled eggs are better than fried eggs in terms of fat quality.

You can have eggs on their own, with fruit on the side, with avocado and tomatoes, or with spinach as Eggs Florentine. If you want to have toast with your eggs, try toast from non-wheat bread as per the suggestions above, or you could have them with oat cakes. Sprinkle herbs, pepper and a little good-quality salt such as sea salt or Himalayan salt over them for taste.

Omelette

If you are partial to an omelette, it makes a good weekend breakfast.

Ingredients (serves one)

½ onion or 2 spring onions
2 tomatoes
½ cup mushrooms
2 organic, free range eggs
Cold-pressed unrefined groundnut or avocado oil (available

from health food shops)
Extra-virgin olive oil for drizzling
Butter (optional)
½ - 1 tablespoon grated organic cheese (optional)
Herbs
Salt and pepper
Pumpernickel, rye, or whole wheat bread

Chop the onions, tomatoes and mushrooms. Heat 1 tablespoon of water in a frying pan. When the water is steaming, add the chopped ingredients (this is the *healthy sauté* method – see Fats Week). Stir over a medium heat until they are cooked. You may also add a small knob of butter.

Transfer the cooked ingredients to a bowl and put them to one side. Beat together the eggs and pour them into the frying pan. If you don't have a non-stick pan, you may need to add a small amount of oil. Groundnut and avocado oils are safest for frying with (see Fats Week), or you can lubricate the pan with a little bit of butter or ghee.

When the eggs are nearly cooked, place the onions, tomato and mushrooms on top. Sprinkle on the herbs and a drizzle of olive oil; you can also add a little organic cheese such as feta or cheddar at this point. Fold the sides of the omelette over the middle and cook for a few more seconds.

Serve the omelette parcel on its own or with a small piece of toast – for a more healthful alternative to toast, try serving it with salad.

Chia jars

Chia jars make a fantastic breakfast because they are very quick and easy to make, and you can make them the night before, so in the morning if you are tired all you have to do is stagger downstairs and eat them, then let their nutrients carry you on a wave of good energy through the morning.

There are many variations on this recipe on the internet, but this is the basic one. A good tip is to stir superfood powders, such as spirulina or acai powder, into the mixture to make it a pretty colour.

You will need a nice large glass jar to use as a container.

Ingredients:

2 tablespoons chia seeds
2-3 tablespoons porridge flakes (eg oats or millet flakes)
1/2 - 1 tablespoon maple syrup or agave syrup (to taste)
1 teaspoon vanilla essence or paste OR 1/2 - 1 teaspoon cinnamon powder
2 tablespoons live plain yoghurt or soy yoghurt, unsweetened
Dairy-free milk such as oat milk, nut milk or soy milk - approx 1 - 1.5 cups
Fresh fruit e.g. berries, bananas, soft fruits such as peaches or apricots
Mixed nuts (optional)

In the evening, put the chia seeds, porridge flakes, yoghurt, maple syrup and vanilla or cinnamon in the jar. Add enough of the milk to cover with an extra cm or two on top (exactly how much depends on the shape of your jar - you want enough liquid for the solids to swell into overnight; the finished texture should resemble that of rice pudding). Give it a really good stir to mix the chia seeds in otherwise they will clump.

Cover and leave overnight at room temperature, then add the fruit and nuts on top in the morning before eating. Keeps for around two days in the fridge.

Black beans

In Costa Rica, including Nicoya, its 'Longevity Hot Spot', ask anyone what they have eaten for breakfast and they are almost certain to have had *gallo pinto* – rice and beans. (They are likely to have had it for lunch and supper, too). *Gallo pinto* means 'spotted rooster', referring to the black and white speckled appearance of the dish. They may also have had some *huevos* – eggs – on the side, as well as a juicy pineapple or mango freshly-fallen from a tree nearby.

Beans are a good source of protein, as well as vitamins, minerals, and fibre, and they make a more sustaining start to the day than toast or cereal. They should be soaked overnight or longer in warm water to reduce anti-nutrients (see Proteins Week). White rice is not good for health (see Carbohydrates Week), so the good health of the Nicoyans must be in spite of, rather than because of, the rice. I suggest using a small amount of quinoa, brown rice or a corn tortilla instead, or you can forego these completely and have the beans with some guacamole and a poached egg.

Cooking beans may seem like a bit of an effort, but you can cook them in a large batch and freeze them in portions, ready to use at any time.

Ingredients for cooked black beans

500g dried black turtle beans, soaked overnight or longer and drained (you can use tinned black beans sometimes as a short cut but these will be lower in nutrients)
1 onion, cut in half
2 garlic cloves, whole
1 organic chicken stock cube dissolved in a little water or 2 teaspoons salt
1 small bunch coriander stems

Put the ingredients in a pan and cover with water so that the water level is around an inch above the ingredients. Bring to the boil, cover, and simmer, stirring occasionally, until the beans are soft. This will take around 1-2 hours, depending how long the beans soaked for. Check the beans from time to time, adding more water if necessary.

The next stage is to make refried beans with your cooked beans:

<u>To make refried beans (serves 2)</u>

Ingredients

2 cups cooked black beans (as above)
1 small onion, chopped
1 clove garlic, minced
1 teaspoon ground cumin
1 organic chicken stock cube
A small knob of butter or ghee (optional)
1 tablespoon extra-virgin olive oil (optional)

To serve

1-2 tablespoons chopped coriander
Soured cream

Heat a tablespoon of water in a frying pan until steaming, with a little chicken stock cube if you want to (the *healthy sauté* method – see Fats Week). Add a little butter or ghee if desired. Add the chopped onion and cumin and cook, stirring, for 5 minutes. Add the garlic and cook for one minute. Add the black beans. Mash them up in the pan with a potato masher, adding a little water or stock if necessary. You want to end up with a kind of lumpy purée. Once you have turned the heat off, add the olive oil and stir in.

Serve with quinoa, brown rice or on a tortilla, garnished with the soured cream and coriander. If you have any leftover black beans from the first stage of cooking, these can be frozen and used another time.

Sprouted bread

Sprouted wheat or rye bread is a dense, moist, filling, low-gluten type of bread made from sprouted wheat or rye grains. It is easier to digest, more sustaining, and higher in nutrients, including protein, than ordinary wheat bread. Sometimes called *Essene* bread, it is available from good health food stores. It is slightly sweet, so goes well with nut butter and fruit spread, or honey. It suits being toasted.

Maple syrup and apple sauce granola

Personally I don't find granola very digestible – it usually leaves me feeling slightly uncomfortable, and it can also be quite sweet. However, I am including this recipe here for granola-lovers, and because it is at least higher in protein and other nutrients than the vast majority of breakfast cereals, as well as being lower in sugar than most shop-bought granola.

Ingredients

2 tablespoons unrefined groundnut oil/walnut oil
125 ml maple syrup
2 tablespoons honey
300g rolled oats/millet flakes/quinoa flakes/multigrain flakes(as desired)
50g sunflower seeds
50g pumpkin seeds
4 tablespoons sesame seeds
100g flaked or roughly chopped almonds
2 teaspoons ground cinnamon
¾ cup unsweetened apple sauce
50g dried fruit (eg raisins, blueberries, cranberries)

Heat the oven to gas mark 2/150C/130 fan. In a large bowl, mix together the solid ingredients apart from the dried fruit. In a saucepan, gently heat the apple sauce, honey, oil, and maple syrup. Add to the dried ingredients and mix well. Spread the mixture on baking sheets and bake for 15 minutes. Add the dried fruit, stir, and bake for a further 15 minutes. If the granola is not cooked to a golden colour, cook for 5-10 more minutes until it is done. Remove from the oven and cool. Serve with yoghurt or soy yoghurt and oat milk or soy milk; you can also add a tablespoonful or two of ground flax seed for extra protein and good fats.

Keeps in an airtight container for one month.

Better breakfast smoothie

As well as eating something more substantial you can try having a smoothie in the morning. Drinking lots of sweet fruit smoothies is not a good idea, because they contain concentrated fruit sugar called fructose. Fructose is thought to cause insulin resistance which can lead to weight gain and diabetes. Fructose also raises levels of harmful fats called triglycerides, and it increases a process called *glycosylation* which speeds up the ageing process in the body.

Fruit juice is usually even higher in fructose than smoothies, and should be avoided, or diluted with plenty of water. Both fruit juice and high-fruit smoothies can damage tooth enamel, and are not popular with dentists.

However, a smoothie with well-chosen ingredients can be a delicious way to bump up your intake of nutrients and start the day off right. Try the following combinations:

- Apple + grapes + celery + lettuce + spinach + cabbage + cucumber + mint + water
- Berries + yoghurt (live plain yoghurt/kefir/soy yoghurt) + oat or soy milk + ground flax seeds
- Banana + yoghurt + ground flax seeds + oat or soy milk
- Avocado + banana + yoghurt + spirulina and/or chlorella + ground flax seeds + oat or soy milk
- Papaya + banana + raw unrefined coconut oil + yoghurt + ground flax seeds + oat or soy milk

Breakfast – in summary:

- Aim to eat breakfast every day
- Include protein and good fats in your breakfast to balance blood sugar levels
- If you are not hungry at breakfast time, wait for an hour and then eat breakfast

My 'human guinea pigs' do Breakfast Week

Claire was in the habit of either missing breakfast or snatching something insubstantial, so she agreed to make an effort to eat breakfast and to make sure to include protein in the form of nuts and seeds or a boiled egg. After Breakfast Week, she said: 'the eating of the breakfast has really helped because there's no way I've snacked like I normally snack and I haven't really eaten rubbish during the day at all. My energy levels were definitely more constant rather than up and down'. Claire confessed that she had had a croissant one morning, but otherwise she made sure to include some form of protein 'and then I was fuller for longer.'

Ollie tended not to eat breakfast, partly because he was eating large suppers fairly late at night and wasn't hungry in the morning, and partly because he felt he didn't have time. Instead he would have several coffees and by mid-morning he would be ravenously hungry and would go out for a snack of pizza or a chocolate bar. He would also have a large lunch of stodgy food, which would usually be followed by an energy crash. During Breakfast Week, Ollie managed to have breakfast – a sugar-free muesli with nuts, seeds and fruit – every day, partly by eating supper earlier the night before and partly by varying his breakfast time. He found that it stopped him from having 'that desperate hunger' mid-morning and he was able to drop the unhealthy snack. He also felt 'more level'. As an added bonus, he found that sitting with his children eating breakfast also felt like a positive thing to do as a father.

2

Fruit Week

Fruit has become, very unfairly, a bit of a *bête noir* recently, and I am often asked 'should I eat fruit?' by people who have read bad things about it in newspapers and on internet sites. It is a shame there is this confusion about fruit, because it is in fact an excellent and delicious source of all kinds of anti-ageing vitamins, minerals and phytochemicals. Our hunter-gatherer ancestors would have eaten plenty of it, as do the Longevity Hot Spot folk, and it is perfectly compatible with human physiology.

The reason people have become suspicious of fruit is because of its content of fruit sugar. We now know that fruit sugar, or fructose, *in excess* belongs firmly in the 'bad for you' category, and is strongly linked with chronic diseases such as heart disease and diabetes. It is good therefore to avoid concentrated sources of fructose such as are found in fruit juice, high-fructose corn syrup, food products with added fructose, and large amounts of dried fruit.

However, the fructose content of whole fruit should not cause any problems with blood sugar, and a piece of fruit or three a day is positively beneficial for health for the vast majority of people. Results from a recent large-scale study indicated that eating more whole fruit is strongly linked with a lower risk of Type 2 diabetes – although note that fruit juice was shown to increase the risk (1). Blueberries, grapes, apples, bananas and grapefruit came out tops where the anti-diabetes effect is concerned.

Some people find they get bloated after fruit, especially certain fruits, which is thought to be due to problems digesting fructose and fibre or other digestive problems. Apples, melons, pears and papayas are some of the fruits which are more likely to cause bloating, whilst berries and citrus fruits tend to be easier to digest. Avoid eating fruit after a heavy meal, as it can ferment in the stomach whilst it 'waits in the queue' to be digested and cause bloating. People with candida may also find that eating fruit causes bloating because of all the fermentation, and may find that avoiding fruit for the first two weeks of an anti-candida diet helps.

Keep dried fruit consumption to a minimum, and, if you crave a lot of fruit, bear in mind that eating huge amounts can be a crafty way of feeding a sugar addiction. Avoid fruit juice or dilute it well with water, not just because it is high in fructose but because it damages tooth enamel.

A good time to eat fruit is in the morning with or before breakfast, or as a mid-morning or mid-afternoon snack. You may find, if you are hungry, that fruit is surprisingly satisfying and provides enough energy to keep you going until the next meal. Aim to eat two or three pieces of fruit daily.

Ten reasons to eat fruit

1. Eating fruit and vegetables regularly is associated with a lower risk of cancer, heart disease, stroke, Alzheimer's disease, cataracts, and functional decline associated with aging (2). It is also associated with lower risk of Type 2 diabetes.

2. Fruit tastes good – the reason it has developed that way over time is to tempt animals and birds into eating it so that the seeds will be dropped somewhere to grow into a new plant.

3. Eating fruit helps keep your skin young because it provides vitamin C, which is necessary for building collagen. Collagen is also used to keep blood vessels strong and supple, which is why sailors' gums used to bleed when they were suffering from scurvy (vitamin C deficiency.)

If your gums bleed when you brush your teeth, you may not just need to floss, you may also need more vitamin C.

4. Eating fruit is a great way to get a range of antioxidant vitamins and other phytochemicals which are linked with disease prevention in several ways. These work synergistically, which means that they have extra power for being in combination with each other.

5. Fruit has an anti-inflammatory effect due to its content of antioxidants.

6. Fruit is alkalizing and therefore helps the body to keep the blood at the correct pH, which is slightly alkaline at between 7.35 and 7.45. An alkalizing diet is linked with better bone health, lower risk of kidney stones and lower blood pressure.

7. Fruit is a good source of potassium which helps keep blood pressure down and maintains the water balance in cells.

8. Eating a piece of fresh fruit can satisfy a sweet craving without causing any detrimental effects.

9. Fruit contains anti-stress magnesium, potassium and vitamin C, which supports our adrenal glands and helps them respond to stress.

10. Fruit contains both soluble and insoluble fibre which helps keep your colon free of the toxins that can lead to bowel cancer. Apples have been found in studies to reduce the risk of colon cancer (3).

11. Some fruit, such as berries, can actually make you brainier, since they contain proanthocyanidins which enhance neuronal pathways and help regenerate nerve cells.

Which fruit?

To avoid getting stuck in a fruit rut, try exploring the fruit aisles of your supermarket or local fruit supplier, visiting local farmers' markets, having a fruit box delivered, or picking your own at fruit farms. Get local, seasonal, organic fruit whenever possible, since it is likely to have been picked when riper and therefore will be both higher in nutrients and contain more flavour, not to mention making a smaller carbon footprint. To remind yourself to eat fruit, try keeping a well-stocked fruit bowl in a conspicuous place, or putting fruit in your lunch or snack box.

Here is a guide to some different types of fruit and their benefits:

Acai berries

The acai (ah-sah-ee) fruit is a small purple berry native to Brazil, usually sold freeze-dried when imported. It is extremely high in antioxidants, with 18,500 ORAC (oxygen radical absorbance capacity) units per 100g. It is recommended that we have 3,500 to 6000 ORAC units daily, so we only need a small handful of acai berries to fill the quota. Do not overdose on acai berries, since super-dosing antioxidants may disrupt the delicate balance of antioxidants and free radicals in our bodies.

Acai berries are thought to aid weight loss by speeding up the burning of fat. They contain fibre, immune-boosting plant sterols and both omega 6 and omega 3 essential fatty acids, and 500 times more vitamin C than oranges. They are also showing promise as an anti-cancer fruit since their extract has been found in to kill cancer cells *in vitro* (4).

Apples

An apple a day has been found in studies to help keep colon cancer, liver cancer, diabetes, heart disease and asthma away (5). Cornell researchers have identified that apples have powerful antioxidant power, inhibit cancer cells, decrease the oxidation of fats, and lower cholesterol (6). Apple peel is especially beneficial and contains anti-tumour, anti-allergenic, anti-inflammatory, and anti-viral substances (7).

Apples are a great source of pectin, a soluble fibre which

helps remove LDL cholesterol from the body, and insoluble fibre which helps rid the gut of toxic matter.

Apricots

Apricots contain high levels of anti-cancer beta-carotene and are also a good source of copper, iron, potassium, and fibre. Apricots and their kernels are credited for much of the famed good health of the long-lived people of Hunza in Pakistan.

Avocados

The avocado was once known by the Aztecs as 'the fertility fruit', and its name derives from the Aztec word *ahuacatl*, meaning 'testicle', a reference to the shape of the fruit. It is beloved of the long-lived Nicoyans of Costa Rica, who eat it daily, sliced or mashed into guacamole.

Avocados are an excellent source of immune-enhancing plant sterols, protein, fibre, the powerful antioxidant glutathione, the eye-protective antioxidant lutein, potassium which lowers blood pressure, and fat-soluble vitamin E which protects our cell membranes and blood vessel health.

Avocados are also a source of all eight 'essential amino acids', making them a 'complete protein' (see Proteins Week), and are also full of fructo-oligo-saccharides, the fibres which encourage 'friendly' bacteria to flourish in our intestines. The 'good' fats in avocados help us to absorb fat-soluble vitamins: eating avocado with a carrot can enable us to absorb the beta-carotene in the carrot up to 13.6 times better (8).

Bananas

Bananas are an excellent source of fructo-oligo-saccharides, fibres which encourage beneficial bacteria to colonise the digestive tract, and the soluble fibre, pectin. They contain phenolic compounds which aid kidney health, and can help prevent stomach ulcers as they act as a natural antacid. They are also a good source of folate, which keeps our DNA healthy. If you have high blood pressure, eating a banana or two daily may help, since their high potassium content is so effective at lowering blood pressure that the FDA now allows banana producers to make claims to that effect.

Berries

Berries are particularly high in potent antioxidants called *anthocyanins* and *proanthocyanidins*, which give them their dark, rich colour. Some of the best are blueberries, cranberries, bilberries, blackberries, elderberries, strawberries, raspberries, mulberries, boysenberries, acai berries, goji berries, blackcurrants and redcurrants.

The antioxidants in berries are both fat-soluble and water-soluble and are therefore able to get into both fatty and watery parts of cells to protect them from free radical damage. Proanthocyanidins can cross the blood-brain barrier which enables them to protect brain cells from damage. Blueberries seem to be particularly beneficial, with studies showing that rats fed blueberries perform better on mental tasks than others (9). The antioxidants in berries can also help to keep arteries clear of oxidised cholesterol, aid weight loss, reduce cholesterol, protect the heart, and lower inflammation (10).

Berries contain ellagic acid which causes cancer cells to self-destruct in a process known as 'apoptosis'. In a study in Japan, rats were given a carcinogen to induce tongue cancer and then given either antioxidants, ellagic acid, or nothing. The rats in the first group had lower cancer rates than those given nothing but those given ellagic acid got *no cancer at all* (11). And recent much-vaunted studies have shown that berries enhance the effect of chemotherapy and that when given berry treatment, patients require lower doses of conventional drugs (12).

Cherries

Cherries are also full of anthocyanins, which give the fruit its rich red colour, as well as ellagic acid, vitamin C, fibre, and a substance called perillyl alcohol (POH) which studies show may help prevent the formation and growth of certain cancers (13).

If you suffer from gout, try eating cherries, since they have been found to significantly reduce the severity of attacks (14). Cherries may also be able to aid sleep, especially if you are jet-lagged, since they are a good source of melatonin which influences our circadian rhythms.

Citrus fruit

Oranges, grapefruit, lemons, limes, and tangerines are known to be good sources of vitamin C. They are also high in potassium, which is good for lowering blood pressure and relieving fluid retention, and folate, necessary for keeping our DNA in good shape and reducing the homocysteine levels which can threaten heart health.

Citrus fruits also have anti-cancer properties. The Health Benefits of Citrus Fruits 2003 Commonwealth Scientific and Industrial Research reviews forty-eight studies revealing protective effects against cancer, especially mouth, throat and stomach cancers.

Grapefruit is great for weight loss, because it is very low on the glycaemic index and it contains the antioxidant naringenin, which is thought to help the liver to break down fat. In a study, obese subjects lost significant amounts of weight when eating grapefruit or drinking grapefruit juice daily and had an improvement in insulin sensitivity and blood sugar levels (15).

Coconuts

The special property of coconuts is their unusual content of medium-chain fatty acids (MCFAs), including lauric acid, which have become a subject of scientific research thanks to their healing powers. The MCFAs in coconut have been found to be especially beneficial for the immune system since they are anti-microbial, anti-fungal, anti-viral and even anti-parasitical. One type of bacteria they kill is *Helicobacter Pylori*, which is linked with stomach ulcers.

Coconuts and their oil also relieve diabetes and pancreatitis, lower cholesterol, improve digestion, reduce inflammation, and have antioxidant power (16 - 18). Coconut oil is also a great beauty product and is used by Pacific Islanders to as a moisturiser and hair conditioner.

Coconut oil is safe to cook with, since it is stable when heated. Avoid hydrogenated or processed coconut oil, which will not confer the same benefits, and choose the pure, natural kind. Try adding a spoonful to smoothies or use it to add flavour to Thai stir-fries or other dishes.

Figs

Figs are a great fruit for keeping your colon walls swept of debris, since they have a high fibre content, and they are known as an effective laxative. They may help lower blood pressure, thanks to their potassium content, and they are a source of calcium and magnesium, so can be beneficial for bone health.

Goji berries

These tangy red raisin-like berries have a long history of use in Chinese medicine and rate up there with acai berries on the ORAC antioxidant scale at 25,300 units – meaning you need just 20 grams (less than a handful) to reach your daily recommended intake of antioxidants.

Goji berries have a high content of phytochemicals including 33 minerals and trace minerals, amino acids, vitamins, essential fatty acids, phytosterols and carotenoids. These nutrients work together and are likely to have protective effects against chronic degenerative disease including heart disease and cancer. One of the carotenoids found in goji berries is zeaxanthin, which is valued because it is concentrated in the retina of the eye and protects it from UV damage and so may help prevent age-related macular degeneration (19).

Grapes

Grapes have special properties which can help keep chronic disease away. As well as the usual fruity benefits, they contain the powerful antioxidant resveratrol. Resveratrol works together with another antioxidant in grapes, quercetin, to prevent the formation of atherosclerotic plaque and lower levels of LDL cholesterol. It also lowers inflammation and improves circulation in the body, including to the brain. Studies also show that resveratrol can prevent cancer initiation and progression, it protects DNA, and it causes cancer cells to self-destruct (20).

Resveratrol is found mainly in the skins and seeds of red grapes, so try to buy organic grapes and avoid peeling them. Red wine contains high concentrations of resveratrol and other antioxidants (for more about this see Week Nine). Raisins, being dried grapes, have similar benefits, but are high in fruit sugar so best eaten in moderation.

Guavas

The guava can perhaps be regarded as the Asian equivalent of the apple, since it has good all-round health benefits. Guavas are particularly rich in soluble fibre, which helps get things moving down the colon, lowers cholesterol levels by removing old bile acids, and binds to and removes toxins from the colon.

Guavas are also high in vitamin C, useful for warding off colds and flu, and they are a great source of folate, which protects heart health by lowering homocysteine levels and helps keep our DNA in good shape. Guavas also provide other valuable antioxidants such as lycopene and beta-carotene.

Kiwi fruit

Kiwi fruit is known for being especially rich in vitamin C. In a study of asthmatic children in Italy, it was found that those eating kiwi and citrus fruit regularly were less likely to suffer from wheezing or night coughing than those with low intake – an effect attributed to the vitamin C content of the fruit (21). Kiwi fruit also contains phytonutrients which protect DNA in human cells from free radical damage, and it provides vitamin E which provides protection to both the fatty and watery parts of cells.

Mangoes

Mangoes contain a spectrum of powerful anti-ageing nutrients. These include vitamin C, fibre, beta-carotene, lycopene, vitamin E, folate, copper, and potassium. Mangoes also contain a substance called lupeol which inhibits prostate and skin cancers in laboratory animals (22).

Melons

Melons are a rich source of potassium, vitamin C, beta carotene, and other antioxidants.

Watermelon is a good source of prostate-protective lycopene, and it also contains arginine which improves circulation by raising levels of nitric oxide - something which is good for circulation to ALL parts of the body, any male readers present might like to note. Arginine has also been found to improve insulin sensitivity in type II diabetics (23).

Papaya

Papaya is a wonderful fruit for the digestion, since it contains papain, an enzyme which helps digest proteins. Papaya is also anti-inflammatory and contains a wide range of beneficial antioxidants and vitamins and minerals including vitamin C, lycopene, beta-carotene, B vitamins, vitamin E, folate, calcium, magnesium and potassium.

Peaches

Grown nowadays in the Mediterranean and Asia, peaches originated in China where they were traditionally regarded as a health food. Peaches are a good source of beta-carotene, vitamin C, lycopene, potassium and fibre.

Pineapples

Pineapples are high in manganese, an important co-factor for various biochemical processes in the body, and vitamin C which protects our immunity. A special property of pineapples is their content of bromelain, a protein-digesting enzymes, which is why the fruit is often used as a meat tenderizer. Bromelain is also thought to lower inflammation, reduce coagulation of the blood and to suppress tumour growth (24).

Plums and prunes

As you can tell by their dark colour, plums and their dried version, prunes, have very high antioxidant content. Some of the antioxidant compounds they contain, called phenols, are especially effective at neutralising one of the most damaging free radicals, the superoxide anion radical. Phenols also help protect the fatty parts of our cells from free radical damage, which is good news for our cell membranes and also our fatty brain cells.

Plums and especially prunes are very high in vitamin C and they are also an excellent source of calcium, magnesium, iron, potassium, copper and manganese. Plums and prunes are perhaps best known for their laxative effect, which is thought to be due to their content of fibre and two compounds called sorbitol and isatin. If you suffer from constipation, try eating two or three prunes in the evening or having a glass of prune juice.

Pomegranates

Pomegranates are extra-high in antioxidants and they have also become the subject of interest for cancer researchers recently thanks to some special properties. Recent studies show that pomegranate extract destroys breast cancer cells, inhibits the metastasis of cancer cells, and slows the growth of lung and prostate cancer cells in mice (25, 26).

Studies also show numerous other health benefits from pomegranate extract. It protects heart health by lowering LDL cholesterol and blood pressure, retards the development of Alzheimer's-type plaques in the brains of mice, prevents cartilage deterioration, and even helps prevent the formation of dental plaque (27-30).

Fruit – in summary:

- **Fruit is an excellent source of anti-ageing compounds and antioxidants**
- **Try to eat two or three pieces of fruit each day**
- **Take fruit to work, keep it in your bag, or keep a fruit bowl well-stocked so that you remember to eat fruit**
- **Eat fruit alone or with a small snack rather than after a large meal**
- **Try to eat local, organic fruit as it will be higher in nutrients, but also enjoy a variety of fruits**

My 'human guinea pigs' do Fruit Week

Claire normally didn't eat fruit as she was worried about its sugar content, but I explained that whole fruit is fine and that she just needs to stay away from fruit juice. Claire saw the irony in the fact that she would avoid fruit but crave something sweet in the afternoon and hit the chocolate cake. So we went shopping for fruit and she filled her basket very enthusiastically with plums, peaches, pears and grapes. She enjoyed eating them that week, apart from at the weekend when she felt ill from her ongoing virus – 'My regime went out the window. But I'm back on it now – back on the good stuff.'

Ollie was already in the habit of eating an apple, banana or tangerine from the children's fruit bowl every day so this week wasn't much of a change for him and he had no problem eating two pieces of fruit each day. By the end of this week, the breakfast routine had also become effortless and Ollie found that he was now always hungry and ready for breakfast in the mornings. He was unable to take any exercise as he usually would this week as his children had been off school with colds, but found 'I didn't feel as rubbish as I would normally when I don't take exercise.'

3

Vegetables Week

This is a very important week in The Stacking Plan – one which can have a major influence on your health. If there is one stand-out factor in the diets of long-lived, ultra-healthy people, it has to be a high consumption of vegetables. Eating plenty of vegetables every day is one of the first things any nutritionist will advise and there are plenty of studies which show a strong link between veg-eating and good health and slower ageing (1). You are very unlikely to enjoy good health without eating plenty of vegetables.

Yet vegetables are frequently neglected and sidelined. Many people seem to forget about them so easily, probably because there are so many other temptations on offer from richer, more addictive foods. This is a pity, because not only do vegetables do us a world of good, but they can also be very delicious, if you give them a chance. For example, what would you rather have for lunch – an indifferent tuna sandwich on its own, or with a big salad which includes, say, avocado, rocket, watercress, roasted red peppers, and julienned carrot, with a garlic and herb dressing?

So, if you don't already love vegetables, this week try to look at them anew, and discover how delicious and satisfying they can actually be. Aim to get them into your diet in abundance. You should start to feel the benefits almost immediately as well as in the long term - better immunity, a spring in your step, healthier blood sugar levels, more balanced hormones, clearer and more glowing skin, improved circulation, happier mood, healthier hair and nails, and weight loss are all potential benefits of eating more vegetables.

You should aim always to fill HALF of your plate with vegetables both at lunch and at dinner. This is the equivalent of about six or seven daily servings, which is a good minimum amount to aim for (the UK and US governments recommend five servings of fruit and veg daily, which can translate into a very minimal amount of vegetables). Instead of the other things taking centre stage and vegetables being an afterthought, as tends to be the case, make it the other way around. You can eat your usual way otherwise for now – just make sure those veg get onto your plate.

If you are not used to eating vegetables, for the first few days you might find it easier for your digestive system and taste buds to adjust if you start by filling a quarter of your plate with vegetables for a day or two, then a third, then finally aiming to fill half the plate. Remember, you are stacking on the good habits, so keep going with the breakfasts and the daily fruit too. By the end of this week, you should be doing three very beneficial things, all working together to give you good health.

Why veg have the edge when it comes to anti-ageing:

1. Vegetables, especially when raw, are a rich source of **anti-ageing fibre** that helps "sweep" your colon clean. That prevents toxins and aged faeces from creating cancerous conditions in the colon—or leaking into the bloodstream to cause damage elsewhere.

2. Vegetables are an excellent source of **antioxidant** vitamins, minerals, and other substances that neutralise aging free radicals responsible for cellular damage. That means, amongst other things, fewer wrinkles.

3. Vegetables contain thousands of other plant chemicals, called **phytochemicals**, that have powerful beneficial effects.

4. Vegetables are thought to help protect our **telomeres**, parts of our chromosomes which are linked with the rate

at which we age (2).

5. Vegetables are **anti-inflammatory**, and so dampen down the inflammation which is caused by an unhealthy diet and lifestyle and which underlies most chronic disease and accelerated ageing.

6. Vegetables have an **alkalising** effect which helps the body to maintain blood at the correct pH level of 7.35-7.45. Alkalising diets are linked with better bone health, lower risk of kidney stones, lower blood pressure and possibly lower risk of cancer and better detoxification. Acidifying diets, on the other hand, put a strain on the body and are linked with ill health.

How to eat vegetables:

•   Try always to fill half, or at the very least a third, of your plate with vegetables and/or salad at your midday and evening meals. Try using vegetable-based recipes and make whatever else you eat more of a side-attraction.

•   Eat a range of colours to get a range of nutrients. Different nutrients work synergistically in that they have a much more powerful effect when combined than alone. Red peppers, purple beetroot, dark green spinach or broccoli, and orange carrots or sweet potatoes can be combined to create an appetising 'rainbow' effect.

•   Try vegetables roasted, stir-fried, in salads, sauteed, steamed, in soups, in casseroles, as crudites with dip . . . they don't have to be boring and boiled.

•   Eat both raw and cooked vegetables, since we need nutrients from both - carrots, for example, contain more fibre when raw, but high levels of antioxidant carotenoids when cooked. You could try having salads at lunch time and cooked vegetables at dinner time in order to get enough of both raw and cooked.

•   Avoid overcooking your vegetables, as taste and nutrients are lost with overcooking for most types. For example, if you are steaming broccoli or green beans, keep them slightly on the crunchy side.

- Steaming is better than boiling, since boiling causes minerals to leach out into the water.
- Try to eat organic, locally-grown vegetables, since they do not contain potentially harmful pesticide residues and are likely to have a higher content of certain vitamins.
- You can use some of the veg-centric recipes in the Recipes section of this book. There are of course also hundreds of veg-friendly cookbooks and internet recipes to choose from.
- Try making a vegetable-based packed lunch to take to the office such as vegetable soup (to heat up at the office or take in a food flask) or a large salad with chicken, beans or fish and an olive oil-based dressing.
- If you are eating at a restaurant, try ordering an extra side order of vegetables or a salad if your main course is a bit deficient in veg.

Vegetables to include regularly:

- All green vegetables
- All salad vegetables such as lettuce, rocket, and other raw veg including sprouts
- Cruciferous vegetables such as cauliflower, cabbage, and broccoli
- Red, green and yellow peppers
- Root vegetables, such as sweet potatoes, turnips, parsnips, squashes, pumpkins and carrots (see Week Five for more on root vegetables)
- Seaweed
- Garlic and onions

Is a potato a vegetable?

A potato is, botanically speaking, a vegetable, but it does not really count as a vegetable in nutrition terms – it would be better described as a 'starchy carb' (see Carbohydrates Week). Sweet potatoes can count as a vegetable, since they boast large amounts of nutrients and are less starchy than ordinary potatoes (see below). Sweet corn does not count as a vegetable either – it's a grain.

What about herbs?

Herbs are not classified as vegetables but they are a fantastic way to add flavour as well as antioxidants and other nutrients to dishes, so use them liberally.

A vegetable A-Z

Artichoke

Long revered by the Greeks and Romans as a culinary delicacy and digestive aid, artichokes are a Mediterranean favourite. Artichokes support liver function because of their content of a compound called silymarin, and they contain cynarin which promotes bile secretion and aids the excretion of cholesterol. They are also high in antioxidants.

How to eat artichokes: boil them and eat with lemon garlic butter or olive oil, stuff them, roast them, or eat the marinated hearts – these also make a great pizza topping. Vignole is a fabulous Italian recipe using artichokes with peas and broad beans.

Asparagus

Another Mediterranean favourite, asparagus is, like artichoke, both a culinary treat and possessed of special health-giving properties. It is highly alkalising, it is rich in folate and potassium, and it contains fructo-oligosaccharides which encourage beneficial bacteria to proliferate in our guts. It is a good source of glutathione, a powerful antioxidant which helps the liver neutralise carcinogens. It can also help with fluid retention, since it contains asparagine, a diuretic which helps rid the body of excess salts.

How to eat asparagus: asparagus is great grilled or steamed and served with lemon garlic butter or olive oil, roasted, in quiches and pasta sauces, or in stir fries.

Beetroot

Beetroot is a heart-protective vegetable thanks to its ability to improve circulation and lower blood pressure. In studies from the London School of Medicine, scientists have found that two glasses of beetroot juice can lower blood pressure enough to make it an effective treatment for those at risk (3). This is because it contains nitric oxide, which makes beetroot a potential aphrodisiac, enhancing circulation to *all* parts of the body. This also makes it a good vegetable for improving sporting performance.

Beetroot also has lots of vitamins and minerals including folic acid, iron, and boron, and contains a highly potent antioxidant, betanene, which gives the purple root its vivid colour.

How to eat beetroot: beetroot can be shredded raw and added to shredded carrot or cucumber to make a salad; boiled, cut and mixed with mayonnaise to make a pink-coloured salad; roasted; and in the classic Russian soup *borscht*. It goes well with smoked salmon, onion and dill, and it also makes a beautiful purple risotto. If you want to use beetroot juice to lower blood pressure and you are currently taking medication, consult your doctor first.

Broccoli

If you only eat one vegetable, a good choice is broccoli as it has so many health benefits. Fibre, folic acid, vitamin C, potassium, calcium, magnesium, and beta-carotene are all there in broccoli to help supply your daily needs.

Broccoli is one of the 'cruciferous' vegetables which also

includes cabbage, cauliflower, pak choi and Brussels sprouts. Cruciferous vegetables are a source of *isothiocyanates* which help eliminate cancer-causing agents from the body, and many studies show that broccoli has the power to prevent cancer (4-6). Broccoli also contains an enzyme which converts estradiol into a safer form, thus helping protect against estrogen-related breast cancer.

How to eat broccoli: this versatile vegetable can be steamed, eaten raw with dips, put in stir fries, or added to salads or soups. Steam for 3-4 minutes only to keep the crunch and flavour and to maximise the content of nutrients including vitamin C and isothiocyanates.

Cabbage

Cabbage, eaten regularly in several Longevity Hot Spots, is another cruciferous vegetable with many health-giving properties and it also contains anti-cancer compounds. In the 1950s, at the height of Cold War fears about a nuclear attack, cabbage was fed to animals which were then exposed to radiation, and it was found that those fed cabbage had significantly lower death rates. Today, cabbage is recommended by some oncologists as a way to minimise the side-effects of radiation treatment for cancer.

Cabbage is a valuable source of vitamin C, with one serving (around half a cup) of raw cabbage providing almost four times more than a glass of fresh orange juice. It is also great for bone health since a serving provides 43 per cent of daily calcium and 34 per cent of daily magnesium requirements. Cabbage can lower cholesterol, since the fibre binds to used bile acids so that they can be excreted; one study showed that cabbage was 17 per cent more effective in reducing cholesterol levels than a popular cholesterol-lowering drug (7). Cabbage also contains glutamine, which is good for digestive tract health.

How to eat cabbage: there are several different types and colours of cabbage so try them all – red cabbage is good in salads or baked with apple and vinegar; green cabbage works well raw, steamed, in stir-fries, and lightly sautéed. The less time it is cooked for, the more powerful the anti-cancer isothiocyanates; avoid microwaving cabbage as this has been found to block its anti-cancer properties. One very good way to eat cabbage is as fermented *sauerkraut* – see Week Eight for more on fermented foods.

Carrots

As shown by their orange colour, carrots are a rich source of beta-carotene, a fat-soluble antioxidant which is converted to vitamin A in the body. Vitamin A is crucial for immunity and reproduction and it also helps protect the cells lining our guts and respiratory systems. It is also important for eye health, which is why carrots are said to help us to see in the dark.

How to eat carrots: cooking carrots increases the beta-carotene availability, so it is a good idea to eat them cooked as well as raw – steamed, mashed with other root veg, stir-fried and roasted are all good. We need fats to absorb beta-carotene so have carrots with olive oil in salads and stews. Buy organic and wash them rather than peeling since much of the nutrient content is just below the skin. Chew raw carrots well to get the most from them as they may not be fully digested otherwise.

Cauliflower

Cauliflower is another cruciferous vegetable and relative of the cabbage. Cauliflower contains anti-cancer isothiocyanates and sulforaphane which help the body to process toxins, it is an excellent source of fibre, it contains antioxidant vitamin C and vitamin K, and it is also a source of omega 3 and omega 6 essential fatty acids. Since all of these substances are anti-inflammatory, and chronic disease is closely related to inflammation, cauliflower is a great anti-aging food to include in your regular diet.

How to eat cauliflower: there is cauliflower cheese, of

course, or try sautéing it in garlic and onions for a dairy-free alternative. Cauliflower makes a great-tasting soup, works well in stir-fries, and can be chopped raw to go with dips. To increase the content of isothiocyanates, cut cauliflower and leave it for five minutes before using.

Courgettes

This classic Mediterranean vegetable is a good source of carotenoids which help protect the gut, lungs and eyes, it is high in fibre, and the seeds contain protein and essential fatty acids. Courgettes are also high in manganese, which helps produce sex hormones.

How to eat courgettes: the skin is where most of the antioxidants are, so buy organic or scrub well and don't peel them. Try them grated or in thin slices raw in salads, oven roasted with herbs, onions and garlic, grilled, sautéed, and in soups and casseroles. Courgettes go well with other Mediterranean vegetables such as tomatoes or aubergines, for those who do not have to avoid the nightshade family.

Garlic

Garlic, once known as 'the stinking rose', is popular in all the Longevity Hot Spots, and was used as a cure-all by Hippocrates and in the Middle Ages to ward off the plague. It was used by the Romans and by the Russian army during World War II to prevent wound infections since it is anti-bacterial, anti-viral, anti-fungal and anti-inflammatory. It is also a traditional remedy for sore throats and colds. Garlic is a true super-food, with twelve antioxidants including the very important selenium and zinc.

Garlic has specific anti-cancer properties, since it stimulates our cancer-fighting natural killer cells and it contains a compound, allicin, which causes cancer cells to 'commit suicide' in a process called apoptosis (8). Garlic is known to be particularly protective against stomach and colon cancers:

a meta-analysis of studies on garlic and cancer found that regular consumption can lower the risk of stomach cancer by 50 per cent and colorectal cancer by 30 per cent (9).

How to eat garlic: garlic can be used in a huge range of savoury dishes from all over the world, cooked or raw. Chinese stir fries, Mexican tortillas, Greek tsatsiki, Japanese miso soup, bread dipped in olive oil, salad dressings, stews, soups, bean and lentil dishes, seafood, game, roast veg, pasta sauce…you name it, you can probably put garlic in it. If you have a cold or traveller's stomach, try chopping up a clove and swallowing it with a glass of water after a meal.

If you are cooking garlic, ideally leave it to stand for ten minutes after chopping as this prevents some of the active compounds from being destroyed by heat.

Green beans

Green beans, or 'French beans', are great for bone health since they are one of the best vegetable sources of vitamin K and, like all green veg, they also contain magnesium and calcium. They are particularly high in fibre, so they help keep the colon walls clean and protect against colon cancer as well as lowering cholesterol levels. They also contain vitamin C and beta-carotene for antioxidant protection, potassium to help prevent fluid retention and folic acid for DNA synthesis. They have a very low glycaemic index rating of 15 and are filling, so they are a good food for helping balance blood sugar and insulin levels, which is one of the most anti-aging things you can do.

How to eat green beans: lightly steam them to retain flavour and antioxidants and toss with lemon, olive oil, garlic and parmesan; slice and add to stir-fries, lightly steam so they are still crunchy and add to salads with black olives, or eat them raw – when young they should be juicy, crunchy and sweet.

Lettuce

Lettuce is a rich source of all kinds of useful vitamins and minerals. It contains magnesium and calcium which are friendly to bones and muscles, including the heart muscle, and which also help promote sleep. Lettuce also contains relaxing, blood-pressure lowering potassium, vitamin C and iron for blood health, beta-carotene, vitamin K, and folic acid. Lettuce is low on the glycaemic index and full of fibre, so helps balance blood sugar levels.

How to eat lettuce: add in generous quantities to salad, and pile it into sandwiches. Choose varieties with richer colours and textures, rather than insipid iceberg lettuces. Romaine lettuce is a good choice, with two cups providing all the vitamin K you need for the day, and half the beta-carotene

Mushrooms

Strictly speaking a fungus rather than a vegetable, mushrooms deserve a mention as some varieties have remarkable health properties. The extra-special types of healing mushrooms are the *maitake*, *shiitake*, and *reishi* varieties.

Maitake mushrooms are named after the Japanese word for 'dancing' since on finding one, Japanese mushroom hunters would traditionally dance for joy at finding their prize. Maitake mushrooms lower blood pressure and blood lipids, they contain X-fraction, a substance which aids insulin use in the body, and they also contain compounds called beta-glucans which can suppress the growth of tumours (10).

Shiitake mushrooms, which are eaten by the famously long-lived Okinawans, are high in anti-cancer vitamin D and a substance called lentinan which boosts immunity and is used in Japan as an anti-tumour medicine.

The reishi mushroom, known in China as 'the plant of immortality', also has immune-boosting properties and is thought to protect heart health. It is also used to treat asthma, respiratory conditions, liver disorders and arthritis. It is antiallergic, anti-inflammatory, anti-viral, anti-bacterial and antioxidant.

How to eat mushrooms: use in stir-fries, noodle dishes, soups and other Oriental dishes with garlic, sesame oil and soy sauce.

Okra

This small green vegetable, said to have been a favourite beauty-inducing food of the Egyptian queen Cleopatra, is often found on the table in Okinawa, boiled or in tempura. It is also, of course, a classic on the subcontinent, where it is known as 'ladyfinger.'

Okra's big selling point is its slimy mucilage which comes out when it is cut. The mucilage is a type of soluble fibre which removes unwanted substances from our guts, slows the absorption of glucose, softens stool to act as a laxative, promotes 'friendly' bacteria, and helps lower cholesterol levels.

In addition, Okra is abundant in vitamin C, vitamin K, beta-carotene, iron and calcium. Okra is perfect for those who wish to lose weight since it is nutritious and filling yet contains only 25 calories per cup.

How to eat okra: use in curries, African-style stews, gumbo, in ratatouille, raw, in tempura, steamed, or fried.

Onions and shallots

Like their cousin garlic, onions are antibacterial, antiviral, antifungal and anti-inflammatory. They are rich in quercetin, an antioxidant which has an anti-histamine effect and has been found in studies to lower blood pressure and to block cancer cell promoters (11, 12). Chinese people eating onions regularly have been found to have significantly lower rates of stomach cancer than others (13).

How to cook onions: use red or white ones, scallions, spring onions and shallots. Slice or chop and add to salads, roast them with other vegetables, and use them as a base for sauces, stir-fries, soups, stews and oven dishes. Avoid over-peeling onions as much of the antioxidant content is near the surface. Raw onions have the greatest health benefits.

Seaweed

This wonderful super-food, beloved of the Japanese and long-lived Okinawans, is one of the most nutrient-rich vegetables there is. Seaweed contains no less than ninety-two nutritional elements including essential fatty acids, vitamins, minerals, and trace elements. Its iodine content boosts thyroid health to keep your metabolism working and so can aid weight loss. It also contains magnesium and calcium for muscle and bone health. The soluble fibre in seaweed helps keep cholesterol levels down and is therefore heart-protective.

Seaweed can even protect against heavy metal toxicity and radiation, since it contains alginic acid which binds to and removes heavy metals such as lead, cadmium and radioactive strontium from the body.

How to eat seaweed: there are several different kinds of seaweed, including kelp, nori and wakame. Try using it in Japanese recipes such as sushi, miso soup, or seaweed salads.

Sweet (bell) peppers

Sweet peppers (known as bell peppers in the US), are exceptionally high in vitamin C as well as being a good source of beta carotene, folic acid, and other vitamins and minerals. The red ones also contain the prostate-protective antioxidant lycopene as well as a range of other antioxidant phytochemicals which help protect our cells from aging free radical damage. Sweet peppers are also an excellent source of cholesterol-lowering, gut-protective fibre.

How to eat sweet peppers: enjoy all the colours – red, green and yellow – sliced raw to make colourful salads and crudités; roasted and skinned; sliced into stir fries; and used in Mediterranean-style stews, soups and pasta sauces. They are also perfect for stuffing with a variety of fillings.

Sweet potatoes

Sweet potatoes, with their juicy orange flesh, are a much better choice nutritionally than white potatoes. They are high in fibre, low in calories, and lower on the glycaemic index than ordinary potatoes, so they can be included in low-carb diets. They contain vitamin E, vitamin C, fibre, and minerals including zinc, copper, magnesium, iron and phosphorus.

Sweet potatoes are richer in beta-carotene than any other vegetable, with one or two sweet potatoes providing all you need for the day. Other orange and yellow vegetables such as pumpkins and squashes are also excellent sources of beta-carotene. Sweet potatoes are recommended by the National Cancer Society as a cancer-preventative food.

How to eat sweet potatoes: Choose organic and eat the skin for extra nutrients and fibre. Bake them, roast them, mash them, sauté them, and use them in soups and casseroles. Eat them with olive oil, since this will increase your absorption of beta-carotene. With beans and salad they make an ultra-nutritious, well-balanced, satisfying and low-calorie meal.

Spinach

Spinach, a staple of Popeye the muscular sailor man, as well as the long-lived people of Hunza in Pakistan, is one of the highest-ranking vegetables in terms of nutrient-richness. It is a good source of fibre, protein and non-heme iron. It also provides magnesium and calcium for bone health, vitamin K for bone health, anti-ageing alpha-lipoic acid, heart-protective folic acid, beta-carotene, and lutein and zeaxanthin for eye health.

How to eat spinach: spinach can be steamed, added to stir-fries, cooked with chopped onion, wilted in a little olive oil, made into soup, put in Greek-style pies, and eaten raw in salads. Boiling spinach in water allows acids to leach out into the water which gives the spinach a sweeter taste. A poached egg over spinach, or eggs Florentine, will give you a double dose of eye-friendly antioxidants lutein and zeaxanthin and is a perfect protein dish.

The iron in spinach is in the non-heme form, which means it is absorbed best when accompanied by vitamin C, so combine it with other vitamin C-rich foods such as cabbage or red peppers. Spinach contains oxalates so if you have kidney problems or gallstones you may need to avoid or restrict it in your diet.

Tomatoes

Tomatoes are technically a fruit, but are included here since they are usually treated culinarily as a vegetable. Tomatoes are eaten copiously in the Mediterranean and are known to be a crucial part of the beneficial traditional diet there.

Tomatoes are the best food source of lycopene, a powerful antioxidant which is thought to help prevent prostate cancer – a cancer which is common in the West but rare in the Mediterranean. One study has shown that tomatoes eaten three to four times weekly appear to reduce the risk of cervical cancer in women by 70 per cent and another study has shown that eating tomatoes regularly may reduce the risk of aggressive prostate cancer by 53 per cent in men (14, 15).

Lycopene also protects cardiovascular health by lowering 'bad' LDL cholesterol levels, with one study showing a huge 65 per cent reduction in heart disease risk for women eating ten servings of tomato products weekly (16).

How to cook tomatoes: if you get vine-ripened tomatoes or other good quality tomatoes which actually taste like a tomato is supposed to taste rather than the flavourless ones which fill the supermarkets, these are great in Greek salads and with avocado and basil. Avoid tinned tomatoes since they contain toxic Bisphenol A – buy tomatoes in jars or cartons instead.

Cooking tomatoes in olive oil raises the lycopene content and availability in the body, so use tomatoes, tomato paste and tomato sauce for pasta sauce, pizza toppings, soups, stews, black beans, dhal, and baked dishes.

Vegetables – in summary:

- Vegetables are high in anti-ageing, anti-disease compounds and are extremely beneficial for health in many ways
- This week, aim to fill half your plate at the midday meal and half your plate at the evening meal with vegetables
- Eat both raw and cooked vegetables for a variety of nutrients
- Eat a range of vegetables for a variety of nutrients
- Try to eat organic, locally-produced vegetables as much as possible

My 'human guinea pigs' do Vegetables Week

Claire was still not over her virus and was craving junk foods as a 'quick fix' as she felt tired and ill, 'but I have to get on with it otherwise I'll never get out of this vicious cycle of never getting better. I know that I need more vegetables – definitely.' This week, she took care to prepare delicious high-vegetable meals, such as butternut squash with roasted garlic and fried cabbage. She said at the end of the week: 'My energy levels are bad and my house looks like a bomb has hit it…but I do think I'd be feeling worse if I wasn't doing this, if I wasn't having the breakfast and the fruit and the vegetables.'

Ollie initially found it hard to get through the mound of rather bland steamed vegetables such as broccoli, cauliflower, cabbage and greens which he heaped onto his plate. He also felt bloated and windy at first – 'my body didn't quite know what had hit it'. However, these symptoms eased off as his body adjusted, and over the following weeks he varied his ways of cooking vegetables and found that he enjoyed both them and their good effects 'more and more'. In general, Ollie found that he had more energy than usual this week, and particularly noticed this during the early evenings when usually he would feel lethargic.

4

Proteins Week

Where protein is concerned, you want to make sure you get enough of it as well as the right kinds of it. This is a very important part of feeding your body what it needs to operate well, and the benefits to you should be far-reaching.

Eating the right amount of protein is crucial for balancing your blood sugar levels because it steadies the release of glucose into the bloodstream. This is fundamental to having good health and slowing the ageing process, as well as having better energy levels and fewer cravings. You should also find that if you can get your proteins right, you will be able to manage your carbs much better, which will help next week, Carbohydrates Week, to slot into place nicely.

Protein foods are our weight-loss friends because protein is satisfying and it also has a high 'thermic effect', meaning that the body spends more calories metabolising protein than with fats or carbohydrates. We also need protein for cell repair, making immune bodies, making hormones, and to provide us with B vitamins which we use for energy, brain chemicals, and other important functions.

This week, therefore, your task is to make sure you get enough protein so as to steady your blood sugar levels and also to choose the right types of protein. Different sources of protein are described in detail in this section to help you choose well. Continue also with what you are already doing from the first three weeks, eating breakfast, fruit, and plenty of vegetables with your midday and evening meals. By the end of this week you should be really starting to feel the good effects.

How much protein do we need?

The US Recommended Daily Allowance for protein is 63g for men and 50g for women aged 25 – 50, or 0.8g per kg of bodyweight daily. This is less than your average heavy meat-and-cheese eater, but corresponds with the amount eaten, on average, by people in the Longevity Hot Spots. More may be needed by people with extra needs, such as bodybuilders or women during pregnancy and lactation. Paleo eaters also eat significantly more protein than this, but with the important proviso that this is as part of a strict Paleo diet containing large amounts of fruit and vegetables, the right fats, and no starchy carbs – so if you wish to make calculations based on Paleo principles, please refer to expert advice from a source such as Dr Loren Cordain's recommendations.

The basic aim of this week is to get you to eat protein *at every meal*, but without eating a lot of fatty meat and cheese. As a rough guide, eat how much of a protein food will fit into the palm of your hand at every meal, or aim to fill one quarter to one third of your plate with a protein food. A moderate-sized piece of fish, a piece of lean meat or chicken, an egg or two, a cup of beans, a handful of nuts and seeds, a few pieces of tofu or some dhal with yoghurt are all good examples.

By now you should already be having a protein with breakfast – if not, use this week to try and get that good habit into place. If you want to have a snack which is more than just a piece of fruit, try and include a protein with your snack rather than going for something sugary.

Protein content of different foods

Use this guide to plan your meals for protein types and content. You can also use it to compare relative protein values – milk, for example, is not as good a source of protein as some people think.

100g serving	Amount of protein provided (g)
Steak	30g
Tuna, salmon, halibut	26g
Chicken	25g
Pork	25g
Cheddar cheese	25g
Mixed nuts	23g
Cod	21g
Amaranth	16g
Quinoa	14g
Buckwheat	13g
Kidney beans	12.5g
Tofu	12g
Black beans	8.7g
Lentils	9g
1 cup milk	8g
2 tbsp peanut butter	8g
1 egg	6g
Low-fat yoghurt	5g

Complete proteins and why we need them

Proteins break down into amino acids, eight of which are *essential amino acids*, meaning that we need to get them every day from our diet in order for our bodies to function optimally. Protein from animals, birds, fish, eggs, and dairy products provide all eight essential amino acids.

Most plant proteins do not provide all eight essential amino acids. However, mixing plant proteins such as nuts or beans with whole grains does provide all eight essential amino acids, so vegetarians and vegans can get all eight easily enough.

Quinoa, soya, and avocados are plant foods which, whilst they do not have the highest protein content, do contain all eight essential amino acids; hemp, buckwheat, amaranth and millet have all eight although not in optimum levels.

Which proteins?

Deciding which proteins to eat can be confusing, because research is ongoing and opinions differ. Heart-friendly Mediterranean diets include protein from fish, beans, nuts and seeds, some poultry and eggs, and a little bit of meat and cheese. Longevity Hot Spot diets are similar. Paleo diets contain more meat and fish than other protein sources, but, crucially, the meat must be from lean, grass-fed animals.

Given that most protein foods have their upsides and downsides, whether nutritional or logistical, my advice is to use the information below to make careful protein choices and to do a bit of experimenting. You may find it suits you best to rotate and vary your protein foods. I also like mixing proteins together – lean minced lamb with aduki beans, for example, chicken in miso soup, or quinoa with tofu and pumpkin seeds; this will help get your protein to the right levels. The main thing is that if you are someone who finds you have better energy levels and fewer cravings after this week, you know you are on the right track with your proteins.

So, here are the high-protein foods, with their main benefits and drawbacks:

Animal proteins

Animal proteins are a mixed bag, and much can depend on how the animals or fish they come from are reared.

Red meat

Red meat is a controversial subject, with 'nay-sayers' and 'yea-sayers' constantly at odds with one another. It is true that red meat IS linked with increased risk of chronic disease, but the overall picture is complex and it is possible that red meat *per se* should not be getting the blame – it is probably more to do with fats and the way meat is farmed as well as what else is eaten with it. At the very least, I would say that however much red meat you eat, it must be organic, free range or wild, lean, and grass-fed, since this makes all the difference to the fat and protein content of red meat, which in turn can make all the difference to your health.

Benefits of eating red meat

- Red meat is a rich source of protein.
- Red meat is a source of complete protein, containing all eight essential amino acids.
- Red meat is a rich source of iron, zinc, and B vitamins.
- Pork (which can be categorised as either red or white meat), is an excellent source of proline and glycine, which help keep connective tissue strong and elastic.
- When lean and pasture-fed, red meat can contain good levels of essential fatty acids as well as a beneficial type of saturated fat called stearic acid (see Fats Week).

Drawbacks of eating red meat

- Two very large recent studies of over 100,000 people followed for up to 28 years showed that eating red meat regularly is linked with increased cancer, cardiovascular disease and general mortality, even when other factors such as smoking habits are controlled for. The risk was slightly higher for processed or cured meat products such as ham, bacon, and hot dogs, but also applied to non-processed red meat such as lamb and beef. Using other proteins instead was associated with a significantly lower risk (1).

- The majority of meat sold today comes from over-fattened grain-fed cattle which have much higher levels of saturated fat in their flesh than the wild, lean meats our hunter-gatherer ancestors ate, and which are still eaten in the Longevity Hot Spots. Organic, lean, grass-fed meat is available, but you have to shop carefully in order to get it. The overly-fatty meat of today may well explain the findings described in the point above.

- Saturated fat in fatty red meat can lead to inflammation, excess production of oestrogen, and inhibition of essential fatty acid use.

- It is disputed as to whether or not red meat raises cholesterol levels. One review of 54 studies suggested that it does not do so provided that it is lean meat which is trimmed of fat (2). It is known that red meat produces a compound in the body called malondialdehyde which is thought to raise levels of oxidised 'bad' LDL cholesterol, but that antioxidants from, for example, a glass of red wine can counteract this (3).

- Processed meats are usually preserved with nitrites and nitrates which are known carcinogens (cancer-causing agents) and are high in sodium which can affect heart health. One review of twenty studies found a link between processed meats and cardiovascular disease but did not

find the same link with unprocessed meats (4).
- Eating red meat regularly has been linked with higher rates of colon cancer (5).
- When cooked on a high heat, red meat produces compounds such as polycyclic aromatic hydrocarbons (PAHs) and heterocyclic aromatic amines (HAAs) which are known carcinogens. Red meat is also high in arachidonic acid which is linked with cancer.
- Excessive intake of heme iron which is found at high levels in red meat is associated with increased risk of cancer and cardiovascular disease (6).
- Red meat is likely to contain antibiotic, hormone and pesticide residues if not organic. Factory meat also contains cancer-causing pollutants called dioxins.

Tips for eating red meat

- If you eat red meat, choose lean, organic cuts from free-range animals which have been grass-fed. Paleo expert Dr Loren Cordain insists that eating red meat is not damaging to health provided that it is this type of meat and that it is accompanied by plenty of vegetables and no starchy carbohydrates.
- Trim the fat off before cooking.
- Use in casseroles and soups and skim excess fat off the top.
- Try to avoid cured meats – if you do eat them, try to find products cured only with salt and not with nitrites and nitrates – but try to avoid very salty products too.
- Slow-roast, boil, stew, and poach rather than barbecuing, frying or grilling, since this generates fewer carcinogenic compounds.
- Boil meat bones to make stock for flavouring soups and other dishes – meat broth contains free amino acids which are good for the health of our guts. This way you can make meat-flavoured stews and casseroles which are low in meat but high in vegetables.

White meat (eg chicken, turkey)

Benefits of eating white meat

- White meat contains all eight essential amino acids.
- White meat is a good source of B vitamins.
- White meat is a good source of coenzyme Q10 (important for heart health).
- Chicken soup when made with the whole carcass is an excellent source of hyaluronic acid which is used to make collagen and helps keep our skin youthful.
- A 2009 study of half a million people from the US National Cancer Institute found that, whilst red meat raised the risk of mortality, a raised intake of white meat was associated with a slightly reduced risk of death (7).

Drawbacks of eating white meat

- White meat, especially when battery-farmed, can be high in saturated fats (think of the amount of fat which oozes out when you roast a chicken).
- White meat contains no fibre and may lead to constipation and an excess of putrefactive bacteria in the colon which is associated with cancer.
- White meat is acid-forming, so when eaten in excess may lead to excess acidity.
- White meat will contain antibiotic, hormone and pesticide residues if not organic.

Tips for eating white meat

- Eat white meat in moderation and keep the emphasis on the vegetables.
- If you roast a chicken, use the carcass to make stock for flavouring soups and other dishes, and the leftover meat to flavour vegetable-based dishes or to make sandwiches and salads.

- Choose good quality, organic birds or cuts from birds; preferably grass-fed as these will have a better ratio of saturated fats to essential fatty acids in their tissues. Game birds such as duck and pheasant, if you can get them, are a good option.
- Use white meat in vegetable-based casseroles and soups and skim excess fat off the top.
- Slow-roast, boil, stew, and 'healthy sauté' (see Fats Week) or stir-fry briefly rather than barbecuing, frying or grilling, since this generates fewer carcinogenic compounds.

Dairy products (milk, cheese, yoghurt)

Benefits of eating dairy products

- Dairy is a complete protein, containing all eight essential amino acids.
- Live plain yoghurt and kefir can be a good source of probiotics (beneficial bacteria).
- Cottage cheese, soured cream and crème fraiche can also be good sources of probiotics.
- Roquefort, a type of blue cheese, is associated with better heart health, thought to be a result of anti-inflammatory factors contained in its mould (8).

Drawbacks of eating dairy products

- High milk consumption has been found in a recent major study of many thousands of people over 20 years to be linked with higher mortality and higher fracture incidence (9). The study highlights the content of D-galactose in milk which is known to promote ageing and ill health in several ways.
- Milk and cheese are acid-forming in the body which means that the body has to remove calcium from bones in order to alkalise the blood (see below). Live plain yoghurt

does not have the same effect.

- Dairy products, whether high-fat or low-fat, and whether from cows, sheep, or goats, contain growth factors such as IGF-1 which, when they operate in the wrong way in the body, are associated with cell proliferation and cancer (10). Breast and prostate cancer rates are highest in countries which consume most dairy, and some experts believe there is a strong link between the two.
- Dairy products can raise blood levels of calcium which in turn lowers levels of all-important vitamin D.
- Dairy products can be high in saturated fat.
- Cheese is usually high in salt which can cause raised blood pressure and fluid retention.
- Cheese is often high in histamines which cause allergic symptoms.
- Non-organic dairy products usually contain hormones and antibiotics as well as highly toxic dioxins.
- Many people are allergic to or intolerant of dairy products, especially people of Mediterranean or Asian origin (see 'Are you allergic to dairy?' below).

Tips for eating dairy products

- Be wary of dairy! Keep amounts to a minimum.
- If you must eat cheese, choose organic, traditionally-fermented varieties rather than processed products which may have unnatural emulsifiers and colour added and are also high in salt.
- Use cheese to accent food rather than having it in large quantities – you can think of it almost as a condiment, rather than a food source.
- If you drink milk at all, choose organic milk from free range animals as this will have a preferable fat content and lower levels of hormones than non-organic milk. Unpasteurized milk is increasing in popularity since many people report finding it easier to digest than pasteurized

milk.

- If you eat yoghurt, choose live plain sugar-free varieties (these contain beneficial probiotics) rather than long-life, sugary varieties – there is a world of difference between the two.

Dairy products – do we need them for bone health?

Dairy products are high in calcium, which is one reason why we are encouraged to eat them. However, large numbers of people in Asia do not consume milk or cheese, and yet they do not have problems with bone density. Meanwhile, milk-drinking populations have high osteoporosis rates. So what is going on?

All animal products including milk and cheese (but not yoghurt) create acid conditions in the body, which causes loss of alkaline minerals such as calcium from bones, since the body is forced to 'borrow' the calcium from the bones in order to buffer the acid. This means that consuming dairy products may actually be bad for bone health, or at the very least, not as good as the dairy industry would have us believe.

The *American Journal of Clinical Nutrition* reported in 2000 after an analysis of 57 studies that there was no evidence to show that consuming dairy products improves bone health and that some studies actually reveal adverse effects (11). Another key study, the Harvard University's Nurses' Health Study, followed 78,000 women over 12 years, and found that those consuming most calcium from dairy foods had *more* broken bones than those who rarely drank milk (12).

We can get calcium from sources other than dairy products – the best are foods which also contain magnesium since this works with calcium for bone and muscle health. Good sources of both are dark green vegetables, seaweed, tofu, figs, and nuts. Studies published in the *American Journal of Clinical Nutrition* show that high consumption of fruits and vegetables have a beneficial impact on bone health (13). Getting regular weight-bearing exercise also helps maintain bone density.

Are you allergic to dairy?

Most Asians, people of African descent, and Mediterranean people are intolerant to lactose, the milk sugar found in dairy products; around 15 per cent of Caucasians are also intolerant. Symptoms include constipation, mucus, diarrhoea, and gas. Lactose is found at high levels in cow's, goat's and sheep's milk, medium levels in crème fraiche and yoghurt, and lower levels in cheese. Butter has negligible amounts.

People who are lactose-intolerant lose the enzyme, lactase, which is required to digest the milk sugar, lactose, after around 2–3 years of age, which suggests that humans were not originally designed to drink milk after weaning age. You don't see any other adult mammal racing around trying to drink from the udders of another species.

Some people are also allergic to casein or other proteins in milk and lack the enzymes to digest them well. Respiratory problems are often a symptom of intolerance to these proteins and eczema could also be linked. Those who are intolerant to cow's milk are sometimes more able to digest goat's and sheep's milk, since the protein content differs slightly and the casein content is higher in cow's milk.

The fact is that human milk is ideally formulated for human babies, whilst cow's milk is perfect for calves, sheep's milk for lambs, and so on. Cow's milk is not ideal for humans, young or old, just as human milk is not ideal for calves. We are different species and we produce different types of milk.

There are plenty of good dairy-free milk products around these days – try oat milk, rice milk, almond milk or soy milk.

Fish

Benefits of eating fish

- Fish is a complete protein containing all eight essential amino acids we need on a daily basis.
- Fish is low in saturated fat.
- Oily fish such as sardines, salmon, anchovies and mackerel are a good source of omega 3 essential fats which are crucial for good health and are largely lacking from the typical Western diet.
- Eating fish regularly has been found to cut the risk of heart disease by over a third and to reduce total mortality by 17 per cent (14). The benefits of eating fish are put down largely to the omega 3 oils present and seem to reduce the risk of a wide range of illness including childhood asthma, dementia, diabetes, inflammatory conditions, heart disease and cancer.
- In Iceland, the large intake of omega 3 fats from oily fish has been largely credited for the extremely low rates of depression in the population, since omega 3 fats are important for neurotransmitter function (15).

Drawbacks of eating fish

- Because of our polluted seas, fish can be high in pollutants, such as mercury, PCBs, and dioxins. Larger fish are more likely to contain pollutants, so limit intake of shark, swordfish, and tuna, especially Bluefin tuna, particularly if you are a pregnant or breastfeeding woman.
- Some research, however, indicates that the benefits of eating fish, especially oily fish, outweigh the risks. A study from the Harvard School of Public Health which looked at levels of omega 3 fats as well as toxins in fish concluded that eating 3-6 ounces of fish weekly reduced the risk of cardiovascular disease by 36 per cent and death from any cause by 17 per cent (16).

Tips for eating fish

- Avoid deep-fried and battered fish and instead have it poached, baked, steamed, sautéed using the 'healthy sauté' method, or raw as sashimi or ceviche.
- Get the freshest fish possible – the less 'fishy' it smells, the fresher it will be.
- Tinned fish is lower in nutrients than fresh fish – for example, tinned tuna has 99 per cent less vitamin A than fresh tuna.
- For the sake of our seas, try to choose fish which is not endangered and not caught by bottom trawl, which destroys the ecosystem and kills countless fish unnecessarily. Look for labels such as 'sustainable' or 'caught by pole and line'.
- Farmed fish and shellfish are often fed a diet high in pollutants and may contain antibiotic and other residues, so try to get sustainably-caught wild fish when you can.
- If you dislike eating fish, you can obtain omega 3 oils from other sources (see Week Six.)

Eggs

Benefits of eating eggs

- Eggs are a complete protein source, with all eight essential fatty acids.
- Eggs are a good source of iron, zinc and B vitamins.
- Eggs contain the antioxidants lutein and zeaxanthin which help protect eye health.
- Eggs are a good source of lipase, which helps us to digest fats, and lecithin, which helps our bodies to process cholesterol.
- Contrary to popular belief, eggs do not raise levels of 'bad' cholesterol in the body or increase the risk of heart disease for the majority of people – a Harvard study of 80,000 nurses showed no adverse effect for nurses eating

an egg daily (17). The exception to this rule is people with Type II diabetes and 'responders' – people for whom eating dietary cholesterol has a marked impact on blood cholesterol – who may need to limit egg intake.

Drawbacks of eating eggs

*   Eating eggs in excess may cause constipation – if this is you, avoid having them daily.
*   Some people are allergic to eggs which may cause problems such as psoriasis or eczema – if you suspect you have a problem, try excluding them from your diet for two weeks, then eat some eggs and watch for symptoms over the next three days (unless of course you are likely to have an extreme allergic reaction in which case avoid eggs completely).

Tips for eating eggs

*   Use free range, organic eggs for higher nutrient content.
*   Try to buy eggs from grass-fed hens rather than grain-fed as they will have a higher content of omega 3 fats.
*   Poach, boil or scramble rather than frying so as to reduce damage to the fats they contain.

Vegetable proteins

Vegetable proteins, namely beans and peas (aka 'legumes'), nuts, seeds, and pseudograins - are theoretically great sources of protein for vegetarians and those wishing to avoid eating too much meat.

The bad news is that these foods (and whole grains too) contain certain *anti-nutrients*, which is inconvenient for us, but can save the plant's life if it puts us off eating it and enables it to reproduce in the soil rather than halfway down our digestive tract, which is why they evolved that way.

The most problematic anti-nutrients are probably *phytates*.

Phytates block the absorption of minerals such as calcium and iron and they also inhibit the digestion of protein. People who eat very large amounts of grains and legumes can end up with mineral deficiencies if they do not prepare legumes and grains well.

The other notable anti-nutrients are *lectins* and *saponins*, which can damage the cells lining the gut and cause gut inflammation and 'Leaky Gut Syndrome', and *protease inhibitors*, which prevent proteins from being digested.

We can cheat nature to a certain extent by preparing these foods in a way that reduces their content of anti-nutrients as far as possible, as has been done in traditional societies for hundreds of years. This means that for many people, their benefits will outweigh their disadvantages. It is important to do this if you eat a lot of these foods – vegans and vegetarians for example who use these as staples should take special care. This reduces the likelihood of suffering any health problems from eating these foods and increases their nutrient value. Some susceptible people cannot tolerate beans or whole grains at all due to gut irritation and may have to avoid them completely.

In the Recipes section of this book I have given some basic information about how to prepare these foods so as to minimise the content of anti-nutrients.

Legumes (beans, peas and lentils)

Benefits of eating legumes

- Legumes are a source of vegetarian protein.
- Legumes are low in saturated fat, but contain some beneficial essential fatty acids.
- Legumes are high in insoluble fibre which is thought to lower the risk of colon cancer (18).
- Legumes are a rich source of antioxidant flavonoids and B vitamins.

- Legumes contain minerals such as zinc, magnesium, calcium and iron.
- Legumes contain phytoestrogens, weak forms of oestrogen which can help balance hormones and are thought to soften the effects of the menopause and possibly reduce the risk of breast cancer.
- Legumes contain *saponins*, compounds with soap-like qualities which can lower cholesterol and have anti-cancer properties. However, saponins also have drawbacks – see below.
- Soy beans have particular benefits – see below for more about this funny old bean.

Drawbacks of eating legumes

- Legumes contain the anti-nutrients *phytates, lectins, saponins,* and *protease inhibitors* so they are best when carefully prepared or, for some people, avoided completely.
- Legumes can cause gas in people who have large populations of certain gut flora because of the high amounts of oligosaccharides they contain which are broken down by methane-producing bacteria in the large intestine. Soaking legumes helps prevent this by breaking down the oligosaccharides.
- In some people, usually of Mediterranean origin, fava or broad beans can cause *favism*, a potentially fatal illness.
- Eating undercooked kidney beans or lima beans can be extremely dangerous due to certain compounds they contain.

Tips for eating legumes

- Soaking, sprouting, fermenting, cooking and pressure cooking are all ways of reducing the anti-nutrients in legumes (see the Recipes section).
- Ensure that beans are always well-cooked.
- Try mashing beans up (as with refried beans) and chewing

them really well – this helps to prevent gas.

- Try making legumes into dips, such as hummus made with chick peas, or other beans cooked and blended with olive oil, garlic and lemon.

Special properties of soy beans

Soy beans are popular in Japan, including in the Longevity Hot Spot, Okinawa, and are also eaten by the long-lived people of Bama in China. They are a somewhat controversial bean, however, and require a closer look.

Benefits of eating soy

- Soy is thought to be at least partly linked to the low breast cancer rate amongst Asian women (19, 20). Their possible benefit is attributed to their content of phytoestrogens (plant oestrogens), which may help balance mammalian oestrogen levels in women.
- Soy is a complete protein, providing all eight essential amino acids our bodies require on a daily basis.
- Soy contains immune-boosting plant sterols.
- Soy contains both omega 3 and 6 essential fats.
- The isoflavones in soy protect blood vessels; soy also contains argenine which raises levels of nitric oxide which boosts circulation by keeping blood vessels dilated.
- Soy contains both magnesium and calcium which are required for heart, muscle and bone health.
- Miso, a fermented soy product, is one of the few widely-available vegan sources of vitamin B12, a very important vitamin for brain health. Miso has also been found to bind to and remove radioactive heavy metals from the human body and has been widely reported to reduce radiation sickness in those exposed to radiation.

Drawbacks of eating soy

- The mass-produced, processed soy products and soy-based TVP now available in ready meals, meat substitutes, soy protein isolates and energy bars contain anti-nutrients (see above) and oxalates which contribute to kidney stone formation.
- Studies have shown that soy supplements and processed soy products promote breast tumour growth in laboratory animals (21).
- Foods containing soy products from the US are usually made from GM soy which is thought to cause allergies and may pose other hazards to health.
- The isoflavones in processed soy products and infant formula may be harmful to the thyroid gland since they are 'goitregens' – substances which block iodine absorption.

Tips for eating soy

- The drawbacks of eating soy seem to be limited to mass-produced modern soy products, so avoid eating these and stick to traditional fermented Oriental products such as miso, tempeh, tamari soy sauce and tofu or, better still, fermented tofu. For example, soy protein isolate contains 10,600 mg saponins per kg, whilst tofu contains 590 mg per kg.
- If you want to get really adventurous and you have access to them, you can try fermented products such as Korean *cheonggukjang*, Japanese *natto*, or Chinese 'stinky tofu' (I can't claim to have tried any of these. Yet).
- Soy yoghurt is also a fermented product and is therefore more digestible than processed soy products.
- Soy milk and ordinary non-fermented tofu are less indigestible than modern processed soy products but not as digestible as fermented soy products.
- Cooking soy beans with seaweed is thought to improve their digestibility and also increases the nutritional value

of the dish. Cooking soy beans with cumin, fennel or ginger is also reported to improve digestibility and reduce gas.

- Edamame beans, which are immature soy beans, are more digestible than mature beans and are a traditional dish in Japan and China.

Nuts and seeds

Benefits of eating nuts and seeds

- Nuts and seeds are sources of protein, fibre, beneficial plant chemicals called phytosterols, vitamins and minerals.
- Nuts and seeds are rich in heart-protective vitamin E; one study showed that people who eat nuts five times weekly have a 31 per cent lower risk of getting heart disease than those not eating them (22).
- Nuts and seeds contain calcium and magnesium which are good for muscle health, including heart muscle.
- Nuts and seeds providea omega 6 essential fatty acids (see Fats Week).
- Flax seeds (also known as linseed), chia seeds and hemp seeds contain both omega 3 and omega 6 fats.
- Brazil nuts are high in selenium, a powerful anti-cancer antioxidant mineral – you need just two or three Brazil nuts to get the recommended daily amount.
- Do not fear the calorie content of nuts, since their nutrient and protein content should have a beneficial effect on metabolism and eating moderate amounts should not cause weight gain.

Drawbacks of eating nuts and seeds

- Nuts and seeds contain the anti-nutrients, phytates and protease inhibitors (see above).
- Some nuts, especially peanuts (although peanuts are

technically a type of legume), can be powerful allergens.

- Peanut lectin is a protein which is known to cause atherosclerosis. Peanuts, peanut oil and peanut butter should be eaten in small amounts only.

Tips for eating nuts and seeds

- To make nuts and seeds more digestible and to reduce the content of anti-nutrients, try 'activating' them (see the Recipes section).
- Make sure to choose unsalted, raw (or activated) nuts rather than salted, roasted ones.
- Nuts can get mouldy or rancid quickly – buy the freshest you can find, preferably still in their shells, and keep them in an airtight container in a cool dry place.
- Try keeping them in a jar in the kitchen or office to remind you to eat a handful daily.
- Try crushing them in a coffee grinder, or pestle and mortar if you want to exercise your biceps (and patience), and adding them to pancakes, porridge, baked foods, and smoothies.
- Sprinkle 1-2 tablespoons of flax or chia seeds on your granola or oats, over a pancake, or add to a smoothie for a good start to the day.

Pseudograins: quinoa, buckwheat, and amaranth

The 'pseudograins' are a group of foods which resemble grains, and can be used culinarily as grains, but are actually a type of seed. This means that they can be included as a 'protein' food and have earned themselves a place in Proteins Week. The main pseudograins which are widely available are quinoa, buckwheat, and amaranth.

Benefits of eating pseudograins

- Pseudograins are relatively high in protein compared with ordinary grains. For example, quinoa contains around 14g of protein per 100g, whereas rice contains between 2 and 7g. Pasta and oats have comparable total protein levels to pseudograins but are inferior sources of amino acids.
- Pseudograins contain all eight essential amino acids.
- Pseudograins do not contain any gluten.
- Pseudograins are a source of essential fats, B vitamins, fibre, and minerals.

Drawbacks of eating pseudograins

- Pseudograins contain anti-nutrients (see above).

Tips for eating pseudograins

- Soaking, fermenting and sprouting pseudograins before cooking them will help reduce the phytic acid content (see Recipes).
- Quinoa, buckwheat and amaranth can all be bought whole, in flakes, or as flour, which makes them very useful and versatile for using with savoury dishes in place of rice or pasta, in porridge, or in baking.

Proteins – in summary:

- **Try to eat protein with every meal.**
- **Aim for around 50g protein daily if you are a woman and 63g daily if you are a man. Paleo eaters may eat more than this but ensure it is part of a strict Paleo diet.**
- **If you need a snack which is more substantial than fruit, make it a protein snack rather than a sugary one.**
- **Vary your protein sources and mix proteins at meal times to ensure good levels of proteins and amino acids.**
- **Vegetable proteins contain anti-nutrients so should be**

prepared carefully.

- If you eat red meat, avoid battery-farmed fatty meat and instead choose lean, organic meat from grass-fed animals.
- If you eat soy products, avoid mass-produced processed products and include only traditionally-fermented ones.
- If you suffer from digestive issues such as an inflamed gut or if you have Leaky Gut Syndrome you may need to avoid vegetable proteins – I recommend that you seek expert advice on this subject.

My human guinea pigs do Proteins Week

Claire greeted me at the end of this week with the words 'I'm a quinoa convert!' She found that adding protein to her meals made them much more satisfying so she was able to eat less, volume-wise, and she didn't crave carbs as she normally would. She struggled slightly with eating more expensive food than usual, but 'I've done my best on the funds I have and I haven't done too badly at all.' She included beans, eggs, tofu, pine nuts, a tiny bit of blue cheese, and occasional meat in her meals as protein sources. She also used quinoa instead of rice, finding its higher protein content made it much more sustaining and enabled her to eat less. This week Claire said she was definitely feeling better as a result of her improved eating habits.

Ollie started to notice much better energy levels this week, especially in the evenings when before he would have been lethargic. This made him more active and he liked that 'my children don't have such a tired grumpy dad at the end of the day.' Adding protein also reduced his cravings for refined carbohydrates such as pies and pasties. He included quinoa, fish, eggs, seeds, and beans in his meals, as well as red meat on one day, and he also added nuts to his breakfast muesli which he found enabled him to go through till lunch time without needing a snack. For lunch he would make a salad to have at home or at work and added a boiled egg or quinoa and avocado, and for supper he made vegetable soup and added beans. He snacked on nuts during the day rather than sugary foods if he felt peckish.

5

Carbohydrates Week

Carb Confusion

These days, the word 'carbohydrate' often brings on a conflicting mixture of suspicion, pleasure, and guilt, usually for good reason. Ask more closely, however, and a lot of people don't really know much about carbs. Which ones are good? Which ones are bad? Or are they all bad? Or all good? What even *is* a carbohydrate? The aim of this week, therefore, is to help you get clear about your carbs – and to know which ones to steer clear of.

First, what is carbohydrate? Roughly speaking, carbohydrates are thought of as being foods which are rich either in starch or sugar, both of which are made up largely of glucose. Potatoes, rice, flour products such as pastries and pasta, and sugar itself are the main carbohydrate foods which provide us with a lot of glucose.

Some carbohydates should be eaten minimally or not at all, whereas others may be a useful addition to a balanced diet. Whether or not certain carbs cause problems for you may be partly down to individual digestive systems. I have come to view carbs in the same way that I view technology – they are hard to avoid, they are enjoyable, and they may have some benefits, but they should be used judiciously. Have them as an adjunct, rather than a main attraction.

Your task this week is to familiarise yourself with the different types of carbohydrate foods so as to choose your carbs wisely. You should also continue with what you have been doing for the previous four weeks. This means that around half your plate at your midday and evening meal will contain vegetables and the rest of the plate will either contain protein foods or it will be divided between proteins and carbs.

If you are a strict Paleo eater or you want to try Paleo eating, you may choose not to eat most starchy carbs. Alternatively, if you are a fan of 'food combining', and wish to separate your starches from your proteins, it is best to have a protein food at the midday meal and a carbohydrate at the evening meal, since eating carbohydrate foods in the evening increases levels of serotonin which can aid sleep. There is more about food combining in Digestion Week.

Refined carbohydrates: the worst carbs

The worst carbohydrates are REFINED carbohydrates. These are grains or starchy foods which have had their outer fibrous coating removed. For example, whole wheat is turned into white refined flour, brown rice is turned into white rice, potatoes have their skin removed, and sugar is extracted from sugar cane. This means that the carbohydrate is broken down into glucose quickly in your digestive system, as there is no fibre present to slow the process down, and the result is too much glucose entering your bloodstream too quickly. For this reason, refined carbohydrates are very high on the Glycaemic Index, a measure of how quickly they release glucose into the bloodstream.

Another problem with refined carbohydrates is that the outer skin or husk is where the vitamins and minerals are, whereas the inside is mainly just starch. Since our bodies need those vitamins and minerals in order to process food and turn it into energy, if the carbohydrate doesn't provide them they have to borrow stores from the body, leaving us with even lower levels. This is why refined carbohydrates are known as 'nutrient robbers'.

Refined carbohydrate foods such as biscuits or *pain au chocolat* look so *friendly* that it's easy to ignore the fact that these carbs cause mass death, but they do. If over-eaten, which they often are, they are a prime cause of blood sugar and insulin disorders, obesity, high blood pressure, high triglyceride levels, and inflammation, which are some of the key factors underlying diseases such as cancer and cardiovascular disease (1). They are also responsible for raising levels of ageing free radicals, stimulating cancer cell growth, stiffened collagen, wrinkled skin, and low levels of the 'youth hormone' DHEA.

The good news is that by balancing blood sugar levels – one of the main aims of The Stacking Plan - health problems caused by eating too many refined carbohydrates and sugars can be controlled and even reversed.

Complex carbohydrates – the complicated carbs

The less-bad, but rather complicated, carbohydrates are COMPLEX carbohydrates. As a rule, these are grains or starchy plant foods with their skin or husk still on, such as a whole wheat grain, a brown rice grain, or a potato with its skin on. Vegetables, incidentally, are technically complex carbohydrates, but they are covered in Vegetables Week and we have no issues with those, so I am leaving them out of this section.

Digesting the fibrous part of a complex carbohydrate such as a grain of wheat or rice takes time, so the glucose is released more slowly and blood sugar levels do not swing so wildly. Another way in which these carbohydrates are superior to their refined counterparts is that the outer part of the grain or potato is where the vitamins and minerals are. I am dividing complex carbohydrates into grains and root vegetables here, as they behave differently in the body:

Whole grains

Whole grains, because they contain fibre, vitamins, and minerals, are a better option than refined grains. One study, for example, showed that replacing refined grains with whole grains such as porridge oats can reduce the risk of stroke as effectively as taking blood pressure-lowering drugs (2). Another three-year study of post-menopausal women published in the *American Heart Journal* found that eating whole grains such as brown rice slowed the progression of atherosclerosis (3).

However, grains, especially those containing gluten such as wheat, rye, and barley can be hard to digest and can cause damage to the gut lining in susceptible people, which can lead to serious illness such as autoimmune disease. Like legumes, grains contain phytates and lectins, with gluten being one of the most damaging types of lectin. We have only been eating grains for a tiny part of evolutionary history (around 10,000 years), and they do not fully suit our digestive systems – even those that do not contain any gluten, such as rice, can be problematic.

Wheat is the most difficult grain to digest for most, since it contains the harshest form of gluten, known as *gliadin*. People with coeliac disease, wheat allergy, or gluten sensitivity should avoid wheat. Rye and barley should also be avoided by those with coeliac disease and possibly by others. Oats contain gluten, but in a more digestible form which can be tolerated by some people with coeliac disease.

Studies show that thirty per cent of people who do not have coeliac disease have antibodies to gluten in their stool. If you suspect you are intolerant to wheat, try cutting it out of your diet for two weeks, then eating a good amount of it over a day or two. Watch out for symptoms over the next *three* days such as bloating, gas, irritability or tiredness. If you have any of these, you should find that removing wheat from your diet makes you feel much better. You can also try this useful (and free) test with rye and barley.

Whole grains, being a high-carbohydrate food, are also relatively high on the Glycaemic Index compared with vegetables, fats, and proteins, so eaten in excess they can still cause blood sugar and insulin issues. They do not fill us up in the satisfactory way that vegetables, proteins and fats do, so eating them can cause us to eat more calories than we need. Furthermore, the lectins they contain can cause 'leptin resistance', in which we stop responding to the hormone, leptin, which signals when we are full. Whole grains can, therefore, make us put on weight.

I recommend eating grains only in small quantities if at all, especially if they contain gluten. If you have the time and inclination, it is also best to prepare them by soaking and fermenting them to minimise the anti-nutrient content (see the Recipes section for details). If you look at traditional ways of cooking, including some of the methods used in the Longevity Hot Spots, grains tend to be soaked, fermented and sprouted.

For more on grains, please see the guide below.

Root vegetables

Root vegetables are starchy carbohydrates, but they do not bring with them the same potential problems as grains. In the UK, they are a winter staple, and can be a good source of local, organic produce.

Potatoes are probably the most commonly-eaten root vegetable in the UK. They are not the highest in nutrients, and they are a member of the nightshade family (along with tomatoes and aubergines) which means that they can cause gut inflammation in some. They are also relatively high on the Glycaemic Index, especially when they come in the form of crisps or chips. On the other hand, the skin of a potato contains fibre, as well as sixty different phytochemicals, including vitamin C and heart-protective vitamin B6. Therefore, if you eat potatoes, eat the skin too, but try only to eat organic potatoes, since potato skins tend to collect pesticide residues from the soil they sit in.

Other root vegetables such as sweet potatoes, squashes, beetroot, turnips, parsnips, celeriac and carrots are all quite starchy. However, they are valuable sources of nutrients, they are less starchy than potatoes, and they tend to register medium or low on the glycaemic index rather than high. Some can also be categorised just as 'vegetables' and are even included in Paleo recipes. Therefore, I think that if you are including some starchy carbs in your diet, root vegetables are a good option. Root vegetables are wonderful in winter roasts, stews and soups so I have included some recipes for those in the Recipes section.

Pseudograins: quinoa, buckwheat and amaranth

The pseudograins were covered in Proteins Week, but must be mentioned here because they also have a relatively high carbohydrate content and can be used in cooking in place of grains. They are gluten-free and higher in protein than most grains.

A guide to grains

This list of grains and their descriptions is not intended as a celebration of grains or to encourage you to eat a lot of them, but so that you can differentiate between them and identify which are most likely to cause digestive problems.

Whole wheat

Whole wheat contains more nutrients and fibre than refined wheat, but it also contains gluten in its most problematic form (see above).

If you want to and can eat whole wheat without problems, beware of 'brown bread' which can just be white bread coloured brown, and try to get the best-quality whole-wheat bread you can find. If you have time, you might even like to try making your own (see the Recipes section of this book).

Sprouted wheat bread, also known as *Essene* bread, and sourdough bread are more digestible than ordinary wheat bread because the sprouting and fermenting processes reduce phytates and gluten content and free up nutrients so that they are more easily absorbed in the body. Sprouted wheat bread is yeast-free, so suitable for people with candida.

Durum wheat

Pasta is made from durum wheat, a type of hard wheat which is also used to make certain types of bread, such as flatbread and some pizza dough. It is lower on the Glycaemic Index than ordinary wheat, including ordinary whole wheat, but it is higher in gluten. Pasta can be made from either refined or whole durum wheat.

Spelt

Spelt is similar to wheat, but is a more ancient grain. It does contain gluten, but a slightly lower amount than wheat, and some people who cannot tolerate modern wheat do not have problems with spelt, although many do. It is higher in B vitamins, protein and iron than ordinary wheat. It can be used in place of ordinary wheat flour for baking, although it does not rise as high due to its lower gluten content.

Kamut

This is another ancient type of wheat whose name comes from the ancient Egyptian word for 'wheat'. It is more 'natural' than modern wheat in that it has not been engineered and it is also lower in gluten; many people who cannot tolerate ordinary wheat find kamut more digestible. Kamut is also richer than ordinary wheat in protein, vitamins and minerals. Kamut flour makes a good substitute for ordinary flour in baking. The kernels can also be cooked similarly to rice or sprouted.

Barley

Barley is another ancient grain which somewhat resembles rice and is a good accompaniment for casseroles or in place of rice. It can also be found roasted and ground in health food shops as a healthful coffee substitute.

Barley contains B vitamins, calcium and potassium, and it has a more balanced protein content than wheat. Use beige 'pot barley' rather than white pearl barley, since pearl barley has most of the germ and endosperm removed. Barley contains gluten.

Rye

Rye is a source of manganese, B vitamins and anti-cancer selenium, and is also high in fibre. It contains gluten, but this is a weaker form of gluten than the gluten in wheat, which makes rye more digestible for some. Rye is also lower than wheat on the Glycaemic Index. It makes excellent Russian-style sourdough bread and is also used for German-style pumpernickel bread and rye crackers.

Oats

Oats are high in both soluble and insoluble fibre which means they help keep the colon clear of toxins and lower levels of 'bad' LDL cholesterol by scouring out old cholesterol-containing bile acids. One form of soluble fibre they contain, beta-glucan, is particularly effective at lowering cholesterol levels.

Oats contain gluten, but of all the gluten grains their form of gluten is the least problematic for human digestion, so many wheat-intolerant people and even some with coeliac disease can eat oats. They are a good source of B vitamins, vitamin E, and omega 6 essential fats.

Brown rice

Brown rice contains fibre, magnesium, iron, manganese, anti-cancer selenium, and B vitamins, as well as other nutrients, and most varieties are lower on the Glycaemic Index than white rice.

Red rice

This is another type of whole grain rice which has a red husk. It is rich in flavour, texture and colour. It is a good source of B vitamins, iron, calcium, fibre, and antioxidant anthocyanins.

Black rice

Also known as *forbidden rice*, this full-flavoured grain has a black husk and will turn purple with cooking. Black rice is a good source of fibre, iron, amino acids and some B vitamins. Black rice is also very high in antioxidant anthocyanins, hence its rich colour. One study, published in the *Journal of Nutrition*, showed that rabbits fed black rice had 50 per cent lower levels of atherosclerotic plaque than rabbits fed white rice (4).

Corn

Corn can be eaten on the cob, as kernels, as polenta, as corn pasta, and it can also be used to make tortillas. In South America, and in the Longevity Hot Spot, Nicoya, corn is soaked in a solution of calcium hydroxide and then simmered for several hours before being turned into tortilla dough. This process makes the corn much easier on the digestion than ordinary corn and adds calcium; cooking for a long time is also known to liberate antioxidants and anti-cancer ferulic acid from corn (5, 6). Corn flour which has been treated in this way is known as *masa* and is available in the US and the UK in some specialist outlets.

Millet

Millet is unlike other grains in that it has an alkalising effect on the body, which helps offset acidifying meats and starches. It is also a good source of amino acids, B vitamins, minerals, and silicon, a part of collagen.

Millet can be boiled and eaten in the same way as rice, or you can buy it as flakes to add to porridge or as flour for use in baking. Adding it to oats to make porridge or pancakes will increase the nutrient content of your breakfast (see Breakfast Week).

Carbohydrates – in summary:

- **Your plate at the midday and evening meal should be half-filled with vegetables, and the rest may contain either just protein foods or can be divided between a protein food and a carbohydrate**
- **The exception to this is if you practise food combining and you wish to have just a carbohydrate food at the evening meal**
- **The worst carbohydrates are refined carbohydrates – sugar, white flour, and white rice**
- **Whole grains have some health benefits but can cause digestive problems and other health issues**
- **Gluten-containing grains should be avoided by people with gluten sensitivity**
- **Gluten-free grains and pseudo-grains are best when prepared properly**
- **Root vegetables may be a valuable addition to a balanced diet and are more digestible than grains**

My human guinea pigs do Carbohydrates Week

Claire was roasting organic sweet potatoes with garlic to go with some lamb when I checked up on her mid-week, and it looked and smelt 'lush', as she said – 'you can smell the goodness.' Claire was not finding it difficult to incorporate all the elements so far from The Stacking Plan into her diet and she was enjoying her food. She noticed this week that she was having fewer cravings than usual - 'I haven't been feeling as hungry, at all'. She was also no longer constipated. 'Now I'm consciously eating healthier I can see I've regulated myself again without using laxatives or anything nasty like that.' Overall she was feeling 'better than I was before – MUCH better.'

Ollie added sweet potatoes and root vegetables to his meals this week as a replacement for his usual white flour products. When the family did eat rice, he mixed the usual white rice with brown rice so that the children did not notice or complain. He also swapped his usual wheat bread sandwich for a piece of rye bread with his lunch (although when he also gave this up during Drinks Week, he seemed to feel better for it). His main glitch was when he had deep-fried battered fish and chips with work mates for lunch and 'felt absolutely awful until I went to bed' as a result. Otherwise, Ollie continued to feel more energetic for most of the day and the evening, and noticed that he was relying on coffee less.

Since Ollie has no scales in his house he did not know at this point whether or not he had lost any weight, 'but although weight has always been the main focus of any diet I have done in the past, because I am feeling very energised by what I am eating it feels less important at the moment.'

6

Fats Week

If you want to avoid heart disease, cancer, and other degenerative illnesses, if you would like to have glossy hair and velvety skin, and if you would like to be at the right weight for you, then you need to get your fat facts straight. Eating the right fats is absolutely fundamental to avoiding chronic disease and feeling and looking good. Eating the wrong ones – as so many of us do – is a major factor underlying chronic disease and accelerated ageing.

The good news is that the health-giving fats and oils are all out there for us to use – we just have to know which ones they are and how to use them. Adding this to what you are already doing from the previous five weeks will greatly enhance the benefits of your good new habits and should have far-reaching benefits for your health.

Essential fatty acids – the fats which are essential for good health

If you want to enjoy optimum health, it is crucial that you get enough essential fatty acids - also known as *essential fats* - which comprise *omega 3* and *omega 6* fats. Essential fats are also known as *polyunsaturated fats* - but these range from healthful to deadly, depending on how they are processed and where you buy them.

In their fresh, unspoiled state, essential fats keep skin and hair youthful and soft, and our cell membranes also need them for flexibility and to be in the right condition to let nutrients in and toxins out. Essential fats also support immune function, hormone function, mental function, and gut health, they are anti-inflammatory, they improve metabolism, they help balance blood sugar, they reduce blood coagulation, and they can even kill cancer cells (1).

We know that essential fats are linked with a lower risk of diseases of ageing such as heart disease and cancer. One recent study of over 3,000 women, for example, found that those consuming omega 3 essential fats had a 25 per cent reduced risk of breast cancer and reduced risk of all-cause mortality (2).

Around one third of our total fat intake should consist of essential fats, and we need omega 6 and omega 3 fats in a ratio of around 2:1. Most people eating a modern diet are deficient in both, but with the additional disadvantage of having far too much omega 6 fat in relation to omega 3 fat, which causes omega 3 deficiency symptoms such as dry hair, depression and poor immunity, to name but a few. This is thought by some experts to be a significant factor in the high rates of chronic disease in countries such as the US and the UK.

Sources of essential fats

Here's where to get your omega 6 and omega 3 essential fats from. From this week onwards, try to include some of these foods in your diet daily. It may also be a good idea to take a good-quality supplement (see below).

Oily fish (omega 3)

Oily fish such as sardines, anchovies, mackerel, herring, salmon and tuna are good sources of omega 3 fats. Regular fish-eating is a common feature of healthy populations.

Tuna is less high than the others in omega 3 fats and can be high in mercury, so limit intake and stick to light meat tuna which is lower in mercury than other varieties.

<u>Hemp seeds and their oil</u> (omega 3 and omega 6)

Hemp seeds and their oil provide omega 6 and omega 3 fats in a ratio of 3:1, so these products are an excellent way to get your essential fats although it is probably a good idea to get some additional omega 3 fats on top to bring your total ratio nearer to 2:1. Hemp seeds are eaten in Bama in China daily as part of a dish known as 'Longevity Soup'.

Never heat hemp oil as the essential fats will become damaged and damaging (see below for more about heating oils).

Take 1-2 tablespoonsful daily of either hemp seeds or their cold-pressed oil.

<u>Flax seeds and their oil</u> (omega 3 and omega 6)

Flax seed, also known as linseed, contains omega 6 and omega 3 fats in a ratio of 1:4. As the proportion of omega 3 fats is high, flax seed is useful in the short term to bring omega 3 levels up if they are too low in relation to omega 6 fats, as is usually the case with the modern diet. After a few weeks it is likely that any imbalances will be corrected, and so extra sources of omega 6 fats will need to be included in the diet in the long term.

Cold-pressed flax oil as well as ground and sprouted flax are available in health food shops and are perfect for adding to smoothies and porridge. Never heat flax oil as the essential fats will become damaged, and keep it in a tightly shut container in a cool place, making sure to use it before its 'use by' date. If the oil tastes metallic, it is rancid and should be thrown out.

Take 1-2 tablespoonsful daily of either ground flax or better still, ground sprouted flax, or its cold-pressed oil.

<u>Chia seeds</u>

Chia seeds – whose name comes from the Aztec word, *chian*, meaning 'oily' – are a good source of omega 3 fats and are widely available in health food shop as seeds and ground seeds. Chia seeds can also be sprouted - in the US, Chia Pets, terracotta animals sporting tufts of chia sprouts, are popular.

Walnuts (omega 3 and omega 6)

Walnuts, grown in several of the Longevity Hot Spots, are a great source of omega 3 fats. For this reason they are considered to be good for brain health – some enthusiasts like to point out the fact that walnuts actually resemble brains. Eat them fresh out of the shell for best omega 3 fat quality.

Apricot kernels (omega 6)

The oil found in apricot kernels is high in omega 6 fats. The Longevity Hot Spot, Hunza, is famous for its apricot kernels, and it is this which has made the kernels and their oil a popular health product. Apricot kernels are similar to almonds and their oil has a pleasing marzipan-like taste; they are also available as a nut butter which is a great alternative to peanut butter. As with hemp and flax seed oil, do not heat apricot kernel oil.

Free range eggs (omega 3 and omega 6)

Eggs contain both omega 3 and omega 6 fats, but eggs from battery-farmed chickens are low in omega 3 fats and comparatively high in omega 6 fats. The best eggs to eat are free range organic eggs from hens fed an omega 3-rich diet, such as grass – look out for varieties marked as such on the box.

Grass-fed livestock, poultry and game (omega 3 and omega 6)

Plant foods such as grass contain omega 3 and omega 6 fats, so when animals or birds eat them, the essential fats end up in their flesh. Modern battery-farmed animals, on the other hand, are fattened up with grains which cause the flesh of those animals to be higher in saturated fats and lower in essential fats. Grass-fed animal products are eaten by Paleo eaters and in the Longevity Hot Spots and you may also be able to source them from a good butcher – make sure to avoid produce from animals fed GM (genetically modified) grass, though, which at the time of writing this book is about to be unleashed.

The milk of grass-fed, free range animals also contains lower levels of saturated fats and higher levels of essential fats than the milk from their battery-farmed counterparts.

Soy (omega 3 and omega 6)

Soy and its products such as tofu and cold-pressed soybean oil provide both omega 6 and omega 3 fats in a ratio of 7:1.

Spirulina and chlorella (omega 3 and omega 6)

These are forms of algae which contain both omega 3 and omega 6 fats and are available in powder form which is ideal for mixing into smoothies and juices.

Essential fatty acid supplements

Essential fats are available in supplement form which can be very useful since it can be hard to get enough essential fats from food, unless you eat a very traditional diet.

Essential fat supplements are extracts rather than whole foods, so I am wary of them, since as a rule it is better to get your essential fats from your food if you can. Studies into the effects of essential fat supplements are mixed, and we need to know more before we can be really confident about their benefits. If you decide to take supplements, it is crucial that you get good-quality supplements – remember, you get what you pay for.

I also recommend that you consult a qualified nutritional

therapist both as to whether or not to take supplements and how long to take them for. It may be best to take them for a few weeks or months from time to time so as to keep levels up. Do not take essential fat supplements without first consulting your doctor if you are taking medication, especially blood-thinning medication.

Fish oils (EPA and DHA from omega 3)

These provide the end-products of omega 3 fats which our bodies require, EPA (eicosapentaenoic acid) and DHA (docosahexaenoic acid). However, studies seem to suggest that fish oils do not provide the benefits of omega 3 fats in the way that oily fish do. This could be to do with the quality of the oils used in studies, or it could be to do with the fact that fish oil is best absorbed along with other nutrients in the fish along with protein.

If you are going to use fish oil, make sure you get a really good-quality brand or you may do yourself more harm than good. Cheap cod-liver oil supplements are often rancid; beware anything which smells fishy, is not kept in a cool place, or has a long shelf-life. Make sure also to use purified fish oils – fish tend to store toxins in their fats, so non-purified fish oils can be high in nasty pollutants.

Good-quality fish oils contain around 300mg EPA + DHA per 1000mg.

Krill oil (EPA and DHA from omega 3)

Krill oil is a supplement which provides EPA and DHA which have been found to be more easily absorbed than the omega 3 fats in fish oil, since the fats come in phospholipid form, which is the form they take in our cell membranes. Krill oil is also less likely to go rancid than fish oil, since nature packages it along with an antioxidant called astaxanthin which protects the omega 3 fats present. Look for sustainably-sourced, good-quality brands from clean

Antarctic waters. Some people also prefer krill oil to fish oil because there is no 'fishy repeat.'

We need around 300-500mg EPA plus DHA daily, and 1000mg of krill oil contains between approximately 250 and 300mg of EPA plus DHA.

Borage oil, blackcurrant oil and evening primrose oil (GLA from omega 6)

These can be useful supplements for women with a hormone imbalance since they are a rich source of gamma-linolenic acid (GLA), the end-product of omega 6 fats which are required for balancing feminine hormones. Because of factors such as fatigue or stress or bad diet, some people have systems which are not good at making the conversion from omega 6 fats to GLA, so these supplements can be a good way to bring up levels of GLA.

We need around 150mg GLA daily, which is equivalent to 1500mg evening primrose oil or 750mg borage or blackcurrant oil.

Micellised seed oils (omega 3 and omega 6)

Some superior supplements companies produce mixed essential fatty acids with both omega 3 and omega 6 fats using a mixture of linseed and other oils to create the right ratio in a bioavailable form. This is my preferred form of essential fatty acid supplement since you don't need to worry about calculating ratios and the fats are supposed to be in a well-absorbed form.

How to make sure you get enough omega 3 and omega 6 fats in the correct ratio:

You will have to make your own calculations about how much of each of these essential fatty acids you are getting.

As a rough guide, eating a small handful of seeds or

almonds daily plus oily fish two or three times weekly is a basic minimum.

Adding a tablespoonful of ground flax or hemp seed daily will keep levels of both omega 3 and omega 6 fats up. You can also use a tablespoonful of cold-pressed flax or hemp oil for a similar effect.

You can also take a supplement of both omega 3 and omega 6 essential fats (see above) for a while to get your levels up.

Remember, you want a ratio of around twice as much omega 6 as omega 3 in the long term, but you may need more omega 3 fats initially to address any imbalance.

Monounsaturated fats – the very useful fats

Monounsaturated fats (MUFAs) are 'good' fats which help keep our cells, including our skin cells, strong yet pliant. They also act rather like little 'taxis' in the bloodstream, carrying fat-soluble antioxidants to cells to keep them protected from free radical damage.

MUFAs protect against diseases of ageing in a number of ways. A recent trial showed that consuming MUFAs lowers blood pressure, improves blood cholesterol levels, and reduces the risk of heart disease (3). They also help balance blood sugar and insulin levels, which slows the rate at which we age and helps keep us slim.

The best source of MUFAs is extra-virgin olive oil, which is of course a Mediterranean staple and which is often credited for the low rates of heart disease in parts of the Mediterranean, including several Longevity Hot Spots there.

Olive oil has other benefits apart from its content of MUFAs:
- Olive oil contains oleic acid which has been found to *reverse* heart disease in laboratory animals, according to exciting new research (4).
- Olive oil contains heart-friendly, immune-boosting vitamin E.

- Olive oil is good for gut health since it aids the movement of stool down the intestinal tract.
- Olive oil promotes the secretion of bile which we need to process fats.
- Olive oil contains *polyphenols* which are thought to help protect against heart disease and cancer.

Olive oil is best used cold, since cooking it destroys the delicate polyphenols it contains and may make them toxic. You can use olive oil in cooked dishes by using the 'healthy sauté' method (see below) and then stirring in some olive oil once the heat is off. Olive oil is also perfect for dips, salad dressings, and drizzling over anything you like. Use only extra-virgin olive oil since this is highest in nutrients.

Avocados, macadamia nuts and peanuts and their respective cold-pressed oils are also good sources of monounsaturated fats. Oils from these are safer for heating than other oils (see below for more on which oils to cook with). However, use peanuts and their oil only very sparingly as they contain 'peanut lectins' which are known to cause atherosclerosis.

Saturated fats – the in between fats

Saturated fats are quite a controversial fat, with pro-fat people and anti-fat people all telling us different things about whether or not it's ok to eat them. In my opinion, this is because there are several factors to consider when studying saturated fats which need to be taken in to account but often aren't. So what are the facts about saturated fats?

Saturated fats are those which are hard at room temperature – think of the fat in the grill pan after it has cooled, or a lump of cheese or butter. Or, if you like, the yellow stuff which comes out during a session of liposuction. Saturated fats are found mainly in meat and cheese, as well as in our bodies, to a greater or lesser extent. They are a natural substance and they are an acceptable part of our diet when consumed in small quantities.

The problem is that because of modern animal farming methods, the saturated fat content of meat and dairy products is much higher than it would be if we were eating animals in their natural state. Those of us who eat these products regularly may be getting too much saturated fat in the diet. The saturated fats found in battery-farmed, grain-fed animals are also different in composition to those from lean, grass-fed animals. They contain more damaging types of saturated fats such as palmitic acid and less of a type of saturated fat called stearic acid which is found in lean, grass-fed animals.

It is well-known that saturated fats cause inflammation, which is an important factor in most chronic disease such as heart disease and cancer. These fats also cause stiffening of cell membranes leading to insulin resistance which underlies obesity, diabetes and premature aging. Saturated fats also raise levels of oestrogen and 'bad' LDL cholesterol. Some studies show that high intake of saturated fat is associated with an increased risk of heart disease and cancer (5, 6).

If you eat meat, try to obtain good quality, organic and free range products. Cheese is best kept to a minimum, but the saturated fat content is likely to be preferable if the cheese is from lean, grass-fed, organically-reared animals.

Heated oils – the *damaged*, toxic fats

Heating oils, with a few exceptions, will almost always damage them to a greater or lesser degree. Oils are volatile, and it is easy for their molecular structure to be destroyed.

Heating oils causes the formation of free radicals which cause ageing and disease of our cells. It also destroys nutrients such as vitamin E and other phytochemicals and antioxidants. Polyunsaturated fats in cooking oils easily become rancid when exposed to light and air which causes them to form toxic chemicals such as ozonides, peroxides, hydroperoxides, polymers, hydroperoxyaldehydes and polycyclic aromatic hydrocarbons, all of which damage our cell membranes (7).

According to oils expert Udo Erasmus, when oils are heated above 160 degrees centigrade they start to produce damaging *trans-fats*, and they will produce large amounts of these at 220 degrees centigrade and above. Stove-top frying is usually done at a temperature of 190 degrees centigrade (375 degrees farenheit), which means that even cooking below frying temperature will be damaging (see below for more on trans-fats).

Supermarket cooking oils – RBD and dangerous

Most cooking oils sold in supermarkets contain polyunsaturated fats which have become greatly damaged by processing. With the exception of olive oil, all inexpensive cooking oils have been produced with a technique of RBD (refined, bleached and deodorised). This is true even for many supermarket oils labelled 'cold-pressed', since this refers only to one stage of the manufacturing process.

Putting oils through the RBD process means that they end up far-removed from the natural product they once were. First they are mixed with a corrosive base (usually caustic soda, which we use to unblock drains) which removes beneficial compounds from the oil. Secondly they are bleached, which causes rancidity. Finally they are heated on a high heat in order to remove the unpleasant taste caused by the refining and bleaching. This heating process destroys nutrients and produces free radicals and trans-fats. Oils also become mutagenic at these temperatures since it causes the formation of unnatural molecules.

According to Udo Erasmus, the highly toxic molecules in supermarket oils are far worse than the trans-fats which are now being excluded from foods. They only form one per cent or less of the total oil volume, but Erasmus points out that this equates to between three and six billion trillion molecules. Our body contains around a hundred trillion cells, so from one bottle of oil each of our cells gets six billion damaged molecules. And studies with bacteria suggest that just two molecules per cell are enough to affect our DNA, which, when damaged, can lead to cancer.

So which oils should we buy?

As a rule of thumb, it is best to avoid ordinary supermarket cooking oils such as sunflower oil, canola oil, vegetable oil, and corn oil, as they will almost certainly have been processed using the RBD method. Extra-virgin olive oil is the only good-quality oil you are likely to find on the supermarket shelf.

If you want to buy other types of oils, the best place to find them is from health food shops and other speciality outlets. Avocado oil, peanut oil (also known as ground nut oil), cold-pressed sunflower oil, macadamia nut oil and others can all be bought in unspoiled, unrefined form. They should be in a dark container which needs to be kept tightly-closed in a cool, dark place and they will have a relatively short shelf life. They should have a stronger taste than refined oils. If in doubt, ask the manufacturer.

So how can I fry and roast my food?

Do not worry! You can have the best of both worlds. Not only are there ways of cooking which do not involve using damaged, damaging oils, but you can also make sure you DO get a good intake of healthy oils in your diet. Here's how.

'Healthy sautéing' and roasting

'Healthy sautéing', recommended by nutrition expert George Mateljan, is a simple, delicious way to sauté food without using oil. All you need to do is heat a little water or stock in a frying pan or other pan until it is steaming, and then add whatever you are cooking, such as chopped onions and garlic. I was sceptical at first – it sounded a bit bland – but I have found that it makes the food taste even better, since there is

115

no spoiled cooking oil in there.

This method also works very well for roasted vegetables. Just put your chopped vegetables in an oven dish, add a splash of water or stock, and roast on a moderate heat, turning the veg from time to time. If you are cooking meat, you can use some goose fat, lard, butter, or ghee (see below).

After cooking, you can add some extra virgin olive oil to the dish and stir through. This will bring you all the benefits of the oil with none of the dangers, as well as adding texture and unspoilt taste to your food.

Cook with butter, ghee, or lard

Butter, ghee, goose fat and lard are all stable fats which are not damaged with heat. Lard, or pork fat, has traditionally been used in many of the Longevity Hot Spots in traditional cooking. Butter, ghee and goose fat are high in saturated fats, whilst lard consists mainly of monounsaturated fats, so lard is probably better for health. Buy organic versions from free range animals if possible, since toxins tend to get stored in fatty molecules.

Cook with coconut oil

Unrefined, pure coconut oil is fine to heat with as it is a stable oil. Coconut oil contains mainly saturated fats in the form of medium-chain fatty acids which do not have the same adverse effects on the body as the short-chain fatty acids found in meat and dairy products. It is sometimes called a 'lauric fat' since the 49% medium-chain fatty acids it contains are lauric acid, a substance found in breast milk which has anti-microbial properties. Coconut oil is also a good source of vitamin E.

Use coconut oil for recipes where the taste is appropriate, such as Asian or Caribbean recipes. Stick to good-quality unrefined brands.

<u>A note on 'smoke points'</u>

The 'smoke point' is the temperature at which a fat molecule breaks down. At this point a dark, bad-smelling smoke is emitted, and the oil starts to taste unpleasant. Worse, numerous toxic chemicals are produced.

It is commonly thought that it is safe to cook with oils up to the smoke point. However, damage to oil may begin far below the smoke point (see above on heating PUFAs). Therefore, the smoke point of an oil should not be the only indicator of how high it can be heated. In general, oils should be heated as little as possible or not at all.

Hydrogenated fats and trans- fats – the deadly fats

As a measure of how deadly hydrogenated and trans- fats can be, statistics tell us that the average American eats around 6g of them daily, and one study suggests that eliminating these fats from the North American diet could prevent *200,000* deaths each year! (8).

Hydrogenated fats are fats which have been altered by adding a hydrogen atom to the molecule which gives the food they are being added to a longer shelf life as well as a satisfying chewy texture. Needless to say, they are not compatible with our natural biology.

Partially-hydrogenated oils have their hydrogen atom switched to the other side of the molecule, thus altering their structure and making them incompatible with our biology. Partially hydrogenated fats are a type of *trans- fat*.

Trans-fats are fats which are formed in processed and damaged oils and have been widely used in processed foods. These fats generate harmful free radicals, sabotage our cell membrane structure, raise levels of LDL cholesterol, interfere with essential fat function, interfere with body detoxification systems, interfere with insulin use, and promote inflammation.

117

They are linked with chronic disease such as heart disease and cancer and are increasingly being banned from foods.

Interesterification is a new technique which is replacing hydrogenation as a way to make fats solid or semi-solid and is popular for use in the latest spreads and margarines. Beware of replacing one type of processed food with another though - early studies are suggesting a possible link with heart disease (9).

Fats – in summary:

- **Try to have omega 6 and omega 3 essential fats every day in a ratio of around 2:1 from nuts, seeds and oily fish; flax and hemp seeds and their cold-pressed oils are excellent sources of both and you can also get essential fatty acid supplements.**
- **Try to have monounsaturated fats daily or most days – extra virgin olive oil and avocados are excellent sources.**
- **Restrict your consumption of saturated fats from meat and dairy products - choose lean cuts of meat.**
- **Avoid cheap supermarket oils and be careful when heating oil – choose oils carefully or use the healthy sauté method.**
- **Avoid trans- fats and hydrogenated fats from processed foods.**

My 'human guinea pigs' do Fats Week

Claire incorporated 'good' fats into her diet this week in the form of nuts and seeds and uncooked olive oil and flax seed with her salads, and she also found that she liked the taste of her food cooked using the *healthy sauté* method. Claire also dug out a bottle of flax oil from the back of her cupboard which she didn't like the taste of so I suggested that she make it palatable by mixing it with apple sauce and ground flax seed. At the end of this week, Claire said 'my energy levels are good and my skin is really good and I'm sure that has something to do with the oils.' She was also feeling lighter and more toned and was really enjoying her food: 'my intake of rubbish has gone down massively.'

Ollie used coconut oil to cook pancakes this week which he really enjoyed, and he also made sure to eat plenty of nuts and seeds for omega 6 fats and avocado for monounsaturated fats. He stopped cooking with olive oil and used it raw on salad dressings instead. He also started eating more oily fish such as salmon and mackerel. This week coincided with Christmas for Ollie, but he found that although he was indulging in festive foods and drinks he felt 'pretty good for this time of year – I felt really good on Christmas Day evening, when normally I feel rubbish after eating loads of the wrong stuff.' In general he had more energy, was more active, and was less bloated. He also noticed that he had moved down a trouser size.

7

Digestion Week

If you have got this far, it means that you have completed six weeks of The Stacking Plan. Congratulations!! The main factors of an optimum diet are now covered. Hopefully, you have been able to incorporate most of the elements from these six weeks into your daily eating habits, and are starting to feel and see the difference.

No doubt you have heard Hippocrates' famous words, 'you are what you eat'. This week, remember that you are also *how* you eat. You need to eat your food in a way that will enable your body to actually use it, which means digesting it properly. If you tend to wolf down your food without chewing it or whilst rushing around shouting at the children to get ready for school, as most of us do, this week is for you. We will also look at *how much* to eat this week.

This is a good time to consolidate what you have learned and work at getting into a routine where eating well comes naturally. If you feel things are going smoothly, then this might be a week to browse recipes and increase your culinary repertoire. Or, if the new good habits are falling by the wayside, it is a good opportunity to get back on track.

First of all, here are some ways of helping your digestive system to work well, so you can absorb all the wonderful health-giving nutrients you are now getting from your food:

Chew, breathe, and relax

Digestion starts, not in the stomach, and not even in the mouth, but with the eyes. Look at a plate of red, orange, yellow, light green and dark green vegetables or salad, sprinkled with herbs and drizzled with a sauce or dressing, and accompanied by some fresh baked fish or a succulent casserole. This should get you salivating – in fact, your mouth may be watering even now, just thinking about it. This part of digestion is important, because saliva contains enzymes required to break down carbohydrates and it is also antibacterial and antiviral.

The nose is next. Breathe in the aroma of whatever delicious thing you have made and feel your digestive juices galvanise. Put the first forkful into your mouth, taste the flavours, and chew. Then chew some more, and keep chewing. Chew the food to a pulp if you can. If you are sharing a meal with others, chewing well and timing when you speak may take a bit of practice. If you eat with your children, you may notice that they already chew their food well – we tell our children to hurry up and eat their food, but perhaps it is a good thing that they take their time over it.

Chewing will get your stomach producing hydrochloric acid to break down the food (especially protein) and liberate minerals. Hydrochloric acid production tends to decline with age, stress or ill health, and low hydrochloric acid is a common problem which is often mistakenly treated with antacids which only makes the problem worse. Symptoms of low hydrochloric acid production include bloating, flatulence, acid reflux, an itchy rectum, weak nails, and a sour taste in the mouth.

Well-chewed food is easier to digest because the particles will have a smaller surface area for your stomach's enzymes to work on. The production of stomach acid triggered by chewing will also signal the digestive organs further on down the digestive tract to activate enzymes and secrete juices so that nutrients are properly assimilated into the body where they are needed.

Chewing can help us lose weight without having to reduce portions, since it helps get the message to the satiety centre in the brain that we have enough nutrients which in turn signals our hunger hormones to turn off. Horace Fletcher, the 19th Century American health guru and great proponent of chewing, dubbed 'Fletcherization' by his followers, is reported to have lost an astounding forty-two pounds just by chewing.

Relax as you chew and remember to breathe, as this will enhance the circulation in the digestive areas and help you assimilate the nutrients. In the Longevity Hot Spots, people linger happily over their meals, and relax afterwards rather than rushing up to do some photocopying or load the dishwasher. Try to stay sitting at the table for at least five or ten minutes after eating if you can. If possible, laugh, as this will also relax you and increase your enjoyment of sitting down to a meal.

Eat just enough

Over-eating is bad for digestion and is also a major factor behind accelerated ageing and chronic disease. Here are some useful tips on how to avoid over-eating.

Eat until you are not quite full

In the Longevity Hot Spot, Okinawa, where food is considered one of life's great pleasures, there is a saying, *hara hachi bu*, meaning 'eat until you are only eight parts full.' The health-conscious Okinawans know that overeating can make us ill, and that eating just enough makes us feel good.

Eating too much, particularly of low-nutrient or 'empty calorie' food, speeds up the ageing process in several ways. Putting stress on the digestive organs and causing indigestion is the most obvious effect of regularly over-eating. This means that the body will find it harder to use the nutrients which are put in it.

Because we make 'fuel' for our bodies from food, which is something of a 'dirty' process, just as burning fuel in a car is, over-eating means extra amounts of toxins, especially ageing free radicals, which are harmful to our cells and organs. Over-eating also takes up a huge proportion of available energy in the body, which means there is less energy left over for other important tasks such as repairing cells or fighting illness.

Eating until you are not quite full does not have to mean going hungry, because when you eat, it takes up to twenty minutes for your hormones to send the message up to the 'satiety centre' in your brain that enough food has been eaten. You probably know from experience that if you eat until you are completely full, you are likely to find after a few minutes that you are *uncomfortably* full – a bit stuffed - and indigestion and its bedfellows, wind, discomfort, and acid reflux, may follow. It is best to eat until you are only *just* full, then wait a bit and you should find that you are quite full enough.

Eating just the right amount is a simple concept which can bring you a whole host of benefits. It should help you to feel and look better and age more slowly. And it goes without saying, of course, that it will aid healthy weight loss.

Eat high-nutrient, low-calorie foods

You should find that if you eat a high-nutrient meal, such as a good-sized salad with some lean protein and good fats, and perhaps some complex carbs such as brown rice, it will make you surprisingly full despite being relatively low in calories. This is especially true if you chew it well. Food which is high in fibre and nutrients triggers the gut to let the brain know that enough food has been consumed for the body's needs, so you are less likely to overeat.

Most people find that eating high-nutrient food actually makes them feel far more satisfied and replete than eating, for example, a double cheeseburger and chips (which somehow always leaves us craving a milkshake too). This is in spite of the fact that the double cheeseburger and fries will have many more calories.

There is a solid body of research to show that eating high-nutrient, low-calorie foods can have an enormous impact on health and longevity. In the 1980s, researcher Dr Roy Walford fed a high-nutrient, low-calorie diet to rats in thousands of tests, and showed that three-year-old mice, who would usually be grey and arthritic in their old age, were physically similar to one-year-old mice, whilst rats lived 60 per cent longer than other laboratory rats. Dr Walford also practised the methods on himself and a team of human subjects, and found that certain biological markers showed greatly reduced rates of ageing. Dr Walford's method is known as 'calorie restriction', since keeping calories down to a certain level was a crucial part of the experiment.

I am not suggesting that you practice calorie restriction in the way that Dr Walford and his subjects did, as this is impractical for most people. However, the optimum diet, and the way of eating shown by The Stacking Plan, contains mainly high-nutrient foods which just happen to be lower in calories than less healthy foods, so eating this way can be viewed as a less extreme form of high-nutrient, low-calorie eating.

It is generally recommended that women eat around 1800-2200 calories daily and that men eat around 2200-2800 daily, varying slightly according to energy expenditure or body size. The average person in the UK consumes 3,440 calories daily whilst the average North American totals 3,770 (1). Not only that, but many of these calories are 'empty calories', meaning that they come from food which is almost devoid of any nutrient value (or is positively toxic). By eating The Stacking Plan way, you are doing it the other way around – more nutrients, and fewer calories. As a result you should find you have fewer cravings and better feelings of satiety.

Eat slowly

Most of us know what it's like to gobble our food down to fast and suddenly feel overly-stuffed. Eating slowly means that the brain can receive the message that you are full in time to stop, whereas if you eat quickly you are more likely to overshoot the mark. Chewing food well also helps us to eat less since it makes us eat more slowly and liberates more nutrients.

Take a smaller portion

If you find it hard not to finish everything on your plate, try giving yourself a smaller serving, or using a smaller plate. Not cooking excessive amounts in the first place helps, too. When it's a choice between throwing good food away or eating it when we are already too full, sometimes the latter option seems somehow unavoidable, even if it gives us indigestion. All wrong, but we can blame our mothers for nagging to finish our food when we were children.

Dine like a pauper

It isn't just *what* we eat and *how* we eat – but *when* we eat too. Recent studies on mice have shown that if their eating is restricted to an eight-hour time period, with no snacking late at night, they are healthier and slimmer than other mice. This is the case even when the mice are eating a high-calorie, high-fat diet (2).

You may have found that, since Breakfast Week, you have been eating a substantial breakfast, a good lunch, and a somewhat more modest supper, as opposed to missing breakfast and then eating a lot late at night to compensate. This should not only help you to lose excess weight in the same way that the mice in the above experiment did, but it also helps digestion, since the body doesn't like to multi-task eating and sleeping. If you feel hungry before bed, you can have either have a light snack of something not too rich, or save your hunger for the morning and look forward to satiating it with a hearty breakfast.

Eat less one or two days per week

You may have heard of the '5:2 diet' which has become very popular in the last year or two. I am a big fan of the 5:2 way of eating, having tried it myself and felt the benefits. On the 5:2 diet, for two days a week you eat around 500 calories only, and on the other days you can eat as much as you like. People report, along with consistent weight loss, better energy levels, better mood, and various other health benefits.

The Stacking Plan is perfectly compatible with the 5:2 diet and in fact it can enhance it, since it helps you to eat healthily both on the 5 days and the 2 days, and to reduce cravings. On your 'fast' days, you can eat whatever you like according to the 5:2 diet plan, but I recommend sticking to fruit and vegetables, partly because you can eat more volume-wise without going over your calorie limit, and partly because obviously the benefits will be greater than if you eat, say, a sliver of chocolate brownie. I recommend fruit for breakfast, salad with a tiny bit of dressing for lunch, and soup for supper on 'fast' days.

Recent scientific research supports the idea that intermittent 'fasting' (or, as it actually is, eating much less) may be highly beneficial for health. University of California studies showed that eating just 1050 calories per day for two to four day periods boosts immunity by flipping a 'regenerative switch' which prompts our stem cells to create more white blood cells. This reduces the risk of cancer, since our immune cells mop up diseased, potentially cancerous cells floating around in our bodies; monkeys put on a calorie-restricted diet in studies had *fifty per cent* less cancer than controls (3). Another recent study showed that doing fasting cycles slows the growth of tumours and enhances the effects of chemotherapy (4).

Eating less is also good for digestion. Studies show that eating only a very small amount on certain days, or doing a 'fasting cycle', has a significant effect on our gut bacteria, increasing amounts of the 'good' ones and reducing the 'bad' ones (4). This is excellent for the assimilation of nutrients, since 'good' bacteria do much of this work for us (next week, you will be focussing on getting these valuable allies into your system). Eating less also gives the usually-overworked digestive system a break and allows it to recharge its batteries.

The subject of calorie restriction and intermittent fasting is too large for the scope of this book. Please do not undertake a fast or fasting cycle without consulting a qualified practitioner, especially if you have any medical conditions. See the Resources section at the back of this book for suggested reading.

Combine your food

'Food combining' is a practise in which certain foods are not eaten together. Roughly speaking, fruit is eaten alone, vegetables can be eaten with either starches or proteins, and proteins and starches must be kept separate.

People report enormous benefits to both their digestive and general health when they combine foods. If you want to know more about food combining, there are many books and internet articles on the subject; food combining is also known as the Hay Diet.

If you wish to try food combining, I suggest that you have a protein with vegetables at the midday meal and a starch with vegetables at the evening meal, rather than the other way around, as eating carbohydrates at night raises serotonin levels, which boosts sleep.

Digestion – in summary:

- Digesting your food well will enable your body to make better use of the nutrients in your food
- Try to chew each mouthful to a pulp
- Relax and breathe whilst eating
- Eat just enough and not too much
- Try food combining if you suffer from continued digestive problems

My 'human guinea pigs' do Digestion Week

Claire was confident that she was already a good chewer, but when she started to be conscious of her chewing this week she realised that 'it's really not that easy to consistently really masticate properly, especially if you're out eating – you feel people are looking at you thinking you're some kind of food geek.' However, she 'definitely' chewed more than usual, and found that 'my digestion was much smoother than normal – not so much gurgling and flatulence.' Claire also found that by chewing well and by eating 'the right stuff' she was less likely to overeat, and instead was able to have 'an elegant sufficiency.' Claire was feeling good this week, with good energy levels, and she also said she was 'feeling a lot more in control of what I'm eating…I'm not snacking as much, so when I do have treats I don't feel guilty.'

Ollie was used to gobbling down his food and not chewing it or savouring it, and found this week a challenge. Eating until 'just full' was harder than he thought it would be, especially as this week coincided with the Christmas period, and he found that eating slowly and chewing well required a 'massive conscious effort.' He also noticed, even with the new healthy foods he was eating, that he tended to 'graze without thinking - I've been eating loads of nuts without necessarily being hungry for them.' Ollie had found that it usually took him a week to get into each new habit and hoped that next week he would be able to master the conscious eating habits learned this week.

Other than that, he was feeling good and managing to incorporate the first six weeks of the Plan without much difficulty, finding that he now preferred the more healthy foods. He also noted that he was more satisfied after eating healthy food, that he needed smaller portions, and that he had 'less of that lethargic, full feeling' than previously.

8

Probiotics Week

The latest research shows that we shouldn't really be thinking of ourselves as just 'me'. It would be much more accurate to say 'me and my microbes.' We have vast numbers of organisms, such as bacteria, fungi and simpler organisms, living in and on our bodies – more than we have body cells. And we each have our own unique population of microbes, known as our 'microbiome'.

The microbiome is so important that it has been likened to an additional organ, and, as with other organs, some microbiomes are in a better state than others. Unhealthy microbiomes have been linked with obesity, autoimmune disease, skin disease, eczema, arthritis, urogenital disease, poor immunity, mental illness, poor metabolism, allergies, autism, hormonal imbalances, inflammatory bowel disease, irritable bowel syndrome, and colon cancer, as well as many other health problems (1). A healthy microbiome, on the other hand, will help us to stay well.

The microbe populations in our guts are a very important part of our microbiomes which have a profound effect on our health. In fact, without having the right bacteria and other microbes in your gut, you can't have a healthy digestive tract. And without a healthy digestive tract, you can't have good health. The right microbes are also crucial for our immune systems, since an incredible *eighty five per cent* of our immune system is actually located in our guts, and much of our immunity there is directed by bacteria.

Today it is very common to have *dysbiosis* – too many harmful microbes and not enough of the helpful, 'friendly' ones in our guts. If you eat a diet low in plant foods, have had courses of antibiotics, eat a lot of sugar and meat regularly, drink chlorinated water, have taken oral contraceptive pills, suffer from chronic stress, or drink a lot of alcohol you are likely to have some degree of dysbiosis.

Last week, you worked on digesting your food well. This week, your digestive system will receive the cherry on the cake – 'friendly' bacteria, which will enhance your digestion and general health even more. Aim to get enough 'friendly' bacteria into your system, and to make your body a welcoming place for them so they want to stay there and offer you all the wonderful services they provide.

'Friendly' bacteria are fundamental to good health because they:

- Protect the lining of our intestines so that we digest food well and toxins are kept out of the bloodstream
- Produce anti-tumour, anti-viral and anti-fungal substances
- Help keep our immune systems strong by protecting the many immune cells in our guts – around 85 per cent of our immune systems are located in the gut wall
- Manufacture B vitamins which are essential for energy and other functions
- Manufacture essential fatty acids which are crucial for good health
- Aid absorption of vitamins and minerals so we benefit fully from a good diet
- Transmit signals to the brain via the vagus nerve resulting in good brain function
- Produce enzymes such as protease, lipase and lactase to help us digest food
- Produce butyric acid which builds colon cells to keep the colon healthy
- Destroy *e. coli*, *shigella* and *salmonella* by releasing substances such as lactic acid, hydrogen peroxide and

selective antibiotics
- Repel candida
- Neutralise endotoxins produced in the body
- Neutralize potentially carcinogenic nitrites in the digestive tract
- Aid peristalsis (the movement of the gut muscles for stool elimination)
- Get rid of excess cholesterol by breaking down bile
- Lower inflammation by regulating cytokines

Getting your 'friendly' bacteria

Here are some ways of getting probiotics into your system – and keeping them there.

1. Take probiotic supplements

Probiotic supplements can be a quick way to bump up your levels of 'friendly' bacteria. Look for a good-quality brand with guaranteed viability of the organisms, and remember that you generally get what you pay for. Try taking them for a few weeks and then topping up once or twice a year.

If you take antibiotics, it is important to take probiotics to replace the beneficial bacteria killed by the medicine. Some reports suggest that people who start taking probiotics at the same time as antibiotics are less likely to have stomach upsets both than those not taking them and those who take them after the course of antibiotics has finished. If you take probiotics during a course of antibiotics, take them at least two hours apart so that they have more chance of surviving long enough to do some good.

2. Eat fermented foods

Fermented, or 'living', foods are a popular recent health trend, as well as an ancient culinary custom. Fermented foods are still a part of many traditional diets today, including in all of the Longevity Hot Spots. Eating fermented foods regularly is a better way to get probiotics into your system in the long term than taking supplements because they contain many more strains than probiotic supplements do.

Fermented foods are made by adding beneficial bacteria to the food and then leaving it for a period of time. The bacteria enrich the flavour, prevent the food from spoiling, enhance the nutrient content and make the food more digestible by helping break down starches and proteins.

Try to get some fermented foods into your diet on a regular basis – a small amount each day or a few times a week is a good amount to aim for. Avoid too many dairy products or very salty foods. Sauerkraut and kimchi are great options which can be made at home and are also sold in some good health food shops. I also recommend sprouts and pickled vegetables which aren't too salty.

Some common fermented foods:

Pickled vegetables

Pickled vegetables are marinated in vinegar or salt water which preserves them and causes them to ferment in the presence of beneficial bacteria. Capers, olives, artichokes, mushrooms, beetroot, umeboshi plums, carrots, beetroot and cabbage are all good for pickling. Mass-produced versions are pasteurised after fermenting which kills the beneficial bacteria, so either make your own or buy them from health food shops or specialist delis.

Sauerkraut (pickled cabbage) is easy to make at home. Sauerkraut was allegedly fed by Genghis Khan to his plundering hordes to keep them fit and healthy. Captain Cook also used sauerkraut to prevent his sailors from getting scurvy. If you are adventurous in the kitchen you might also like to try your hand at making Korean-style *kimchi* from a range of vegetables. It adds real zing to salads and cooked dishes – a tablespoonful or two is just the right amount, I find.

Soy products

Traditionally-fermented soy products include miso, tempeh, fermented tofu and traditionally-brewed soy sauce, and most soy yoghurt also contains probiotics. Fermenting soy products not only makes them a source of beneficial bacteria but also makes them much more digestible than modern processed soy products, which are an invention of the West and are not eaten by long-lived Japanese or Chinese populations.

Umeboshi plums

These are small, reddish-purple, wrinkled, salty and very tangy pickled plums containing probiotics which are popular in Japan as a digestive aid and as a cure for hangovers and bad breath. They are very potent, and salty - two or three a week is enough. Look for them in Japanese shops or health food shops.

Sprouted foods

Sprouted beans, grains or seeds such as sprouted alfalfa or sprouted mung beans have been soaked in water which causes them to be broken down by beneficial bacteria, which opens them up and gets them sprouting. Sprouted grains can be made into bread known as 'essene' bread.

The sprouting process greatly increases the content of the vitamins, minerals, amino acids, essential fatty acids and enzymes present in the food. For example, vitamin B2 increases by 2000 per cent, folic acid by 600 per cent and vitamin C by 600 per cent in some sprouted foods. Sprouting also makes grains and beans more digestible (and thus less gas-forming), and reduces the content of anti-nutrients such as phytic acid. Another remarkable property of sprouts is that they contain the nucleic acids RNA and DNA which are necessary for healthy cell division and thus may protect against cancer.

A note of caution: sprouted foods can cause food poisoning,

since the sprouting process can cause any harmful bacteria they are contaminated with to proliferate. Even if you grow your own sprouts at home, if they come from contaminated seeds they may be a health hazard. If in doubt talk to your producer about their source and whether they can be guaranteed to be uncontaminated.

Sourdough bread

Sourdough rye and wheat breads are made with dough which is slowly fermented, usually with a combination of yeast and the probiotic *lactobacillus sanfranciscensis*. These types of bread are much more digestible than modern fast-rising loaves which use industrial yeast and chemical enhancers and additives. In addition, some of the gluten is broken down so it is less likely to cause indigestion in gluten-intolerant people.

Fermented milk products

Fermented milk products have a long history of use across the world and are popular in several of the Longevity Hot Spots. The probiotics they contain break down the milk sugar, lactose, into lactic acid, which makes them a more digestible product than milk. Here are some examples of common fermented milk products:

Yoghurt

The best yoghurt you can buy nowadays is low-fat with a creamy, slightly sweet texture and which has been fermented with *L. bulgaricus* and *S. thermophilus*. Yoghurt which has been pasteurized after the addition of probiotics will not contain live cultures and will not provide the same benefits.

Kefir

Kefir is a fermented milk product originating in the Caucasus. The word kefir (pronounced as in the name 'Keifer') means 'pleasure'. Kefir is tangy like yoghurt, and contains a mix of cultures such as *Saccaromyces kefir*, *Torula kefir*, *Lactobacillus brevis* and *Streptococcus lactis*, amongst others. True kefir has a slightly alcoholic content due to the presence of yeast, which gives it its unique flavour.

Crème fraiche

Crème fraiche is cream which has been soured with bacterial culture. It is thick with a slightly tangy taste and is popular for making sauces in French cuisine.

Cheese

Some cheeses are fermented with the aid of friendly bacteria – these cheeses include feta, parmesan, cottage cheese and pecorino. Cheese is best enjoyed in small quantities only, if at all (see Proteins Week).

3. Eat foods rich in plant fibre

Not only do you want to get probiotics into your gut, but you also want them to hang around and colonise. One way to encourage them to take up residence is by eating plenty of foods rich in plant fibre, since this contains fructo-oligosaccharides (FOS) which friendly bacteria live off.

When researchers analysed the stool of people aged 80-109 years old in the Longevity Hot Spot, Bama in China, they found that it contained significantly more of the probiotic *bifidobacterium* than the stool of elderly Chinese from other districts (2). This was attributed to their intake of fermented foods and their diets rich in plant fibre.

Some foods which are particularly rich in FOS are avocados, bananas, and Jerusalem artichokes.

4. Be kind to your friendly bacteria:

Certain things kill friendly bacteria, leaving space for opportunistic pathogenic bacteria and yeasts to flourish and undermine your health. These include:

- Excessive sugar
- Excessive animal fats
- Stress
- Excess alcohol
- Antibiotics

Try to avoid these, and if you do overindulge/suffer excessively from any of these, make sure to top up your levels of 'friends' with a course of probiotics or extra fermented foods for a while to counteract their effects.

Probiotics – in summary:

- **Having 'friendly' bacteria in our guts is essential for good digestive health and good health**
- **Many of us have dysbiosis in which there are not enough 'friendly' bacteria**
- **Make sure to get probiotics into your system by taking probiotic capsules and/or eating fermented foods**
- **Keep probiotics in your system by eating fibrous plant foods**

My 'human guinea pigs' do Probiotics Week

Claire was already in the habit of taking probiotics ever since her daughter had had a course of antibiotics and she joined her in replenishing her good gut flora. This week, Claire also added dill pickles and sauerkraut to her diet. She suffered from a bad stomach for a day or two after a Chinese takeaway of suspect quality, but said 'I do think I got over it quicker because I was taking acidophilus in the morning than I would have otherwise.'

This week, Claire was busy and stressed in the run-up to Christmas, but was managing to incorporate most elements of the Stacking Plan and 'definitely my energy levels are so much improved because I have had a very busy week and normally I really would be suffering by now, but I'm not and I'm certain that that's because I'm eating better.' Claire also noticed that she felt more in tune with her digestion and in touch with her body and its needs than she used to.

Ollie ordered himself a supply of probiotics to take for the month and he got started on those this week. He also had soy yoghurt containing two probiotic strains. This week, Ollie got to grips better with chewing his food, and he also gave himself smaller helpings and ate more slowly. Not surprisingly, he found that he had less of the 'slightly uncomfortable fullness' than before, and realised that, although he had been eating healthy foods, he had probably been gobbling them. 'I felt really good this week', Ollie said. 'I'm feeling really good in the evenings – I feel active and look for things to do, I feel more 'naturally tired' when it's time to go to sleep, and I'm able to get up earlier.' Ollie also noticed that after taking fairly strenuous exercise, his recovery time was much faster and he was able to exercise the next day where before he would have had to rest his aching muscles.

9

Drinks Week

So, that's the eating part almost done – although the final week, next week is about what NOT to eat. By now, hopefully you are eating many good things, enjoying eating them, digesting them well, and enhancing your gut health with your microbial allies. Hopefully you are also feeling and looking on top form as a result.

But what about what to drink? If you are careful about the liquids which pass your lips, all good. But if you are washing your healthy food down with sugary drinks or lashings of coffee, the wonderful potential effects of your good diet will be undermined. This week, therefore, your task is to think about what you drink. This will be the perfect complement to your new healthy way of eating.

Water – the best drink of all

Water is a kind of 'Cinderella' of drinks – hard-working and invaluable, yet often neglected. Some people are diligent about drinking water, but others only rarely experience the pleasure of a simple glass of fresh, clean, cool, hydrating water.

Without water we would soon be dead. Around 60 per cent of our total body weight consists of water, or should do. We need water for circulation, to transport nutrients into and waste out of cells, and to keep our tissues and organs, especially the brain, which should be 75 per cent water, hydrated. Water is good for weight loss as it is an effective, natural appetite suppressant, and it can also prevent constipation in those who have tried and failed using other methods.

What is the best source of water, now that we don't all

have fresh springs to drink from? Bottled water is problematic because of implications for the environment, whilst tap water contains chlorine and heavy metals which can damage health and don't taste nice. Personally, I recommend investing in a really good-quality water filter jug to remove chlorine and other pollutants. There are sophisticated jug filters available these days which also add antioxidant, alkalising minerals to tap water, as well as reverse osmosis systems which can be installed to improve tap water quality. Some water purification systems ionize the water, making it closer to the natural mountain stream waters found in nature.

Water – tapping the benefits

- We need approximately six to eight glasses of water daily, although this will vary depending on where else you are getting liquids from (fruit and vegetables, for example, contain water, or you may drink a lot of soup or herb tea) and how much you perspire that day.
- If you haven't been in the habit of drinking water, and you don't tend to feel like drinking it, try drinking a few glasses daily and you may soon find that you start to notice your own thirst for it as your body 'remembers' how to be thirsty.
- As a general rule, drink at least one half-ounce per pound of body weight per day; more if you are losing water through, for example, exercise, heat, or breastfeeding.
- A good way to tell how hydrated you are is by checking the colour of your urine. Too yellow means it is too concentrated—but too clear means that it may be too diluted.
- Try keeping a bottle of water near you to sip from throughout the day – you can fill an old glass bottle with water from the water filter if you don't want to buy bottled water.
- Avoid drinking all of your water at once as hyper-

hydration can be very dangerous.

- Water is best absorbed when it is drunk at room temperature.
- Try to drink water mainly away from meals so as not to dilute your digestive juices.

Healing herbal tea

Herbal teas of various kinds are drunk for their health benefits all over the world, including in the Longevity Hot Spots. In Okinawa, people drink copious amounts of turmeric tea, in Hunza tea is made with a herb similar to thyme called 'tumuro', and in Bama in China, ginseng and astragalus tea are popular. These teas and others are all used as traditional remedies and have a range of health properties ranging from heart-protective to mood-balancing.

There is a huge range of herb teas available in the West so there's no need for us to go out and pick the herb with the relevant healing properties from the hillside, pleasurable though that might be. These days, we simply have to read the label and choose one which is good for digestion or energising or relaxing or whatever else we desire for our stressed-out systems. Experiment, stock up on some of your favourites, and keep them in the office and at home.

Green tea

Green tea workers in Japan have long been known to have low rates of cancer, and it has been shown in many studies that drinking four or more cups of strong green tea a day lowers the risk of cancer, particularly cancers of the breast, colon, prostate, lung, skin, bladder, stomach and oesophagus. This is thanks to a powerful antioxidant called epigallocatechin-3-gallate (EGCG) which kills cancer cells and prevents tumour growth (1). EGCG also helps the liver to neutralize carcinogens and has the ability to get into our fatty brain cells and give them antioxidant protection.

141

Green tea contains B vitamins for energy and immunity, E vitamins for heart health, and has more vitamin C than an orange. It reduces levels of 'bad' LDL cholesterol and it is also anti-inflammatory – both green and black tea drinking has been found in studies to lower levels of C-reactive protein, a marker of inflammation closely linked to heart disease (2). Green tea is also antibacterial and antiviral and can help kill *Helicobacter Pylori*. Best of all for some, it can aid weight loss by improving insulin and glucose use and by enhancing fat-burning enzymes in cells.

You can boost the power of green tea by eating foods rich in quercetin, such as apples or onions, at the same time, since research shows that the anti-cancer effects of green tea are greatly enhanced in the presence of quercetin (3).

The best-tasting green tea is the high-grade kind which comes in loose leaves. Put about half a teaspoon of leaves in the bottom of a cup, pour in not-quite-boiling water, relax, and watch the leaves unfold into a beautiful 'tea garden'. It tastes even better if you use the tea leaves again for a second infusion.

Contraindications:

If you feel nauseated after having green tea, this is thought to be because of the combination of polyphenols and caffeine, which can stimulate the production of gastric acid. Try drinking it after a meal so as to avoid any nausea.

If you are pregnant or trying to become pregnant, it may be best to limit your intake of green tea, since EGCG is thought to block an enzyme required to use folic acid in cells. Pregnant women are advised to avoid drinking it during the first trimester and limit intake to one or two cups daily thereafter.

Black tea

Black tea, which is oxidized green tea, is a popular relaxing mid-afternoon drink. It is not as virtuous as green tea, but it does contain beneficial polyphenols which have been found in several studies to lower blood pressure and reduce dangerous triglycerides in the blood, suggesting that drinking moderate amounts of black tea may be good for heart health.

Black tea is higher in caffeine than green tea, lower in antioxidants, and higher in tannins, which block the absorption of non-heme iron. So while it's fine to have a cup of black tea, green tea is likely to be better for health if you are drinking more than one or two cups daily.

Adding even a small amount of milk to black tea negates its beneficial effects, since proteins in both soy milk and cows' milk form complexes with the antioxidants in the tea. Try having it with a squeeze of lemon instead.

Red wine

If you want to drink alcohol, some is less bad than others, and some seems to be positively beneficial. Red wine is well-known for its possible health benefits, and is usually given credit for the 'French Paradox' – the fact that although fatty foods are popular in France, cardiovascular disease rates in red wine-drinking areas are historically low. Recent research shows that when red wine is drunk with red meat, the cholesterol-raising properties of the meat are neutralised (4).

Red wine contains powerful antioxidants, including one called resveratrol. Found in the red-coloured skin of grapes, resveratrol has been found to increase the lifespan of laboratory animals and it also has the power to prevent induced cancer in animals (5). Pinot Noir from New Zealand and Cannonau from Sardinia are especially high in antioxidants.

Red wine may also be able to help prevent Type II diabetes, since polyphenols in red wine have an effect on blood sugar regulation – in one study, a small glass of red wine was found to be as effective as a daily dose of a potent anti-diabetic drug (6).

White wine contains lower levels of resveratrol, whilst rosé wine is often made from both red and white grapes and is therefore likely to have a higher resveratrol content than white wine.

Some studies have shown that wine raises levels of oestrogen and that it may raise the risk of a woman getting breast cancer by about 6 per cent (7). In addition, all types of alcohol are linked with cancer. If you do drink, try always to drink in small to moderate amounts and with a meal. It is also better to buy organic wine which does not contain potentially damaging sulfites. Second best is wine made from organic grapes, which may contain sulfites but should not have pesticide residues.

If you drink wine, drink it in moderation only and with a meal, as they do in the Longevity Hot Spots. Try to have two or three alcohol-free nights weekly, and avoid alcohol if you have any liver conditions.

What not to drink

There is more about this next week, but it goes without saying that sugary drinks, caffeinated drinks and spirits should be kept to a minimum or, preferably, avoided.

Drinks – in summary:

- **Try to drink several glasses of water daily, sipped throughout the day**
- **Include herb tea and green tea; black tea can be drunk in moderation**
- **If you choose to drink alcohol, red wine has some health benefits but drink in moderation only and with a meal**
- **Avoid or restrict sugary drinks, caffeinated drinks and spirits**

My 'human guinea pigs do Drinks Week

Claire didn't have to make too many changes this week, since she was already in the habit of drinking water, coconut water, and herb teas during the day. Her main vice was coffee, but she only had one or two per day. Drinks Week happened during Christmas week, and Claire 'madly' did a bit of a detox over Christmas, avoiding rich foods and her usual tipple, cider. She was ill over Christmas – 'it's every Christmas since my weight went on' – but said she was less ill than she would usually have been, and still managed to stay active. Overall, she said, 'I'm feeling really good! I do feel that if I wasn't more conscious of what I'm eating I would be really fat and ill.'

Ollie had already whittled his eight-a-day coffee habit down to two or three cups daily, but he used this week to get down to just one cup, which he found easy to do, and he found that he really enjoyed and savoured his one cup. Instead of coffee, he drank redbush tea, other herb teas, and water. 'I can feel the water hydrating me and it feels good. Now I see that coffee lifted me but then made me tired, whereas the water gives me proper energy'. Ollie had been in the habit of drinking a couple of beers each night, but had given up before Christmas. This week, if he wanted a drink, he had a glass of red wine with a meal. 'I really appreciate that glass of wine – it's like the coffee.'

Ollie was feeling better than ever this week, and for the first time, he didn't feel dozy after lunch, which he speculated was either due to having less coffee or because he cut out his slice of rye bread at lunchtime and had just vegetables and protein instead. 'I feel massively better – a lot more energetic and more in tune with what my body needs. If I do have a lull in energy, I know what I need to get it back more than I used to. It feels hugely different.'

10

No more S.A.D.

You've done it!!! You have completed nine weeks of the Stacking Plan, and now there is only one factor left, which you may already be on top of.

Hopefully, you are enjoying eating this way and see it as being something you can keep going with indefinitely. If you have a family whose eating habits could be improved, your good habits might rub off on them too.

By now you should be feeling the difference, and seeing for yourself the effects of feeding your body what it needs. Increased energy levels, better mood, good hair, skin and nail quality, fewer coughs and colds and effortless weight loss are all things you should be starting to experience. You should feel these effects more and more as time goes on.

This final week, your task is to familiarise yourself with the foods to limit or avoid. If you are used to craving certain of these foods, you may have found that your tastes have changed and that you want them less. That is part of what The Stacking Plan tries to achieve. If you are still finding that a lot of 'naughty' foods manage to find their way into your day, keep at it, and you should find that they are slowly squeezed out and replaced by other things. Try to focus on what you *can* eat, enjoying your favourite Stacking Plan-friendly dishes, and try not to think too much about what you *can't* eat.

If you do indulge from time to time, don't worry about it or feel guilty. Just aim to eat well most of the time, and if you deviate from time to time, that is fine, so long as you stay mainly on track. At the very least, you are now likely to be aware of what makes you feel good and what makes you feel bad, if you weren't already, so that even if you do overindulge in the wrong things, at least you know what you have to do to feel better.

The S.A.D.

The types of foods which are harmful to health tend to make up a large proportion of the modern diet in the UK and the US, and are known collectively as the S.A.D., or Standard American Diet.

Here is a summary of the most common disease-causing foods and drinks:

Sugar

Sugar is so toxic and potentially deadly that scientists are now advising that there should be health warnings on products containing it. Sugar is highly addictive, it is an anti-nutrient, it disturbs blood sugar levels, it depresses immunity, it depletes magnesium, it creates disease-promoting acid conditions, it stresses the adrenal glands, it promotes candida, and it feeds cancer cells. It also raises levels of ghrelin, the 'hunger hormone', leading to over-eating and excess weight.

Beware also of high-fructose corn syrup (HFCS) which is harmful to health because concentrated fructose feeds cancer cells, causes insulin resistance, and can cause diarrhoea in children; HFCS has also been linked with autism since it raises levels of neurotoxins in the brain (1). HFCS also depletes the body of important minerals such as calcium.

Instead: if you crave a sugary snack, eat a protein food to help balance blood sugar levels. Instead of sugar, try whole fruit, stevia, xylitol, maple syrup, good brands of agave syrup and honey as sweeteners instead of table sugar, in limited amounts. If you want to eat chocolate, go for 70% cocoa dark chocolate instead of high-sugar chocolate bars.

Avoid artificial sweeteners such as aspartame as these are

linked with a range of health conditions. New research also shows that drinking diet drinks containing aspartame or saccharine alters the metabolism and disturbs gut bacteria causing a rise in blood sugar levels, which leads to weight gain.

White flour products and white rice

Refined grains such as these cause the release of excessive amounts of glucose into the bloodstream, leading to blood sugar swings, weight gain, cravings, hormone imbalances and lowered immunity. They are also 'nutrient-robbers' which deplete the body of nutrients required to process them. They are devoid of fibre and so can cause constipation and toxicity, and they create acid conditions in the body.

Instead: if you want to eat starchy carbs, avoid refined grains and choose whole grains and pseudograins instead, as featured in Carbohydrates Week.

Deep-fried food

Food which is deep-fried in oil such as chips, crisps, samosas, battered fish, deep-fried chicken, and deep-fried doughnuts, is cooked in damaged cooking oils high in toxic molecules which are linked with heart disease and cancer.

Instead: Try baking, slow-roasting, steaming, stir-frying, stewing, healthy sautéing, or grilling on a low heat instead, and add uncooked olive oil afterwards. Restrict processed foods which have been deep-fried or contain batter.

Processed foods

'Processed foods' include cured meats such as sausages, ham, hot dogs and salami, ready meals, processed cheese, tinned foods, or any foods which have been much altered from their natural state. They often contain additives, large amounts of salt and/ or sugar, trans-fats, preservatives and, in the US, genetically modified organisms (GMOs) and are usually low in fibre and nutrients. Cured meats almost always contain nitrites which form cancer-causing compounds in the stomach.

Instead: try to eat whole foods which require you to prepare them yourself or select processed foods made by a health-conscious producer.

Salt in excess

Excess sodium from salt disturbs the sodium/potassium balance in cells causing fluid retention and Tissue Damage Syndrome (TDS) and it is also linked with high blood pressure, kidney disease, osteoporosis, blood sugar imbalance and stomach cancer (2).

Instead: most sodium needs can be met by eating natural foods which contain a good balance of sodium and potassium. If you must add salt choose unrefined salt such as sea salt which contains minerals or a low sodium brand and use sparingly. Use lemon juice, garlic, herbs and spices to flavour food instead.

Alcohol in excess

Alcohol is toxic to the liver; most alcoholic drinks are also high in sugar. Alcohol is conclusively linked with cancer, it can damage the gut lining, and it kills 'friendly' bacteria. Spirits such as whisky and vodka are particularly high in alcohol.

Instead: restrict alcohol intake; red wine is best as it contains antioxidants and may even be beneficial in small amounts. Choose organic if possible to avoid sulfites and pesticide residues. Try always to drink with a meal rather than on an empty stomach.

Coffee

Coffee is high in caffeine which causes blood sugar swings, it contributes to high blood pressure, it is acidifying, it is linked with migraines and it contains anti-nutrients which cause it to greatly reduce the amount of micronutrients absorbed with a meal (3).

Instead: You can wean yourself off coffee by replacing it gradually with tea, then green tea and/or redbush tea. If you want a comforting hot brown drink, try a coffee substitute such as roasted barley or chicory with hot oat or soya milk.

Carbonated drinks

Carbonated drinks are often high in sugar, additives, and caffeine. They are linked with osteoporosis due to their content of phosphoric acid, and they also cause blood sugar swings. And, according to a recent study from Harvard, drinking just one sugary soft drink a day may raise the risk of having a heart attack by as much as twenty per cent (4).

Instead: replace soft drinks with thirst-quenching water as well as herb teas, green tea, and sometimes vegetables juices and/or smoothies if desired. If you want to drink fruit juice, always dilute it with plenty of water so as to avoid concentrated fruit sugar which is proven to be damaging to health.

Tobacco products

Smokers have a one in two chance of dying an unpleasant, premature death! Smoking is currently the leading preventable cause of death in the US and the UK.

Instead: eating a good diet can help prevent cravings for stimulants. Other methods include self-help books, therapy, and hypnotherapy.

A last word from my 'human guinea pigs'

I am happy to say that neither Claire nor Ollie had any real dietary vices left at this point in the Plan. They had both managed to marginalise their bad habits without feeling that they were being deprived. Both were also enjoying their new way of eating and feeling the benefits. Ollie also discovered, when he weighed himself for the first time since before starting the plan, that he had lost an entire stone in weight.

Claire ate some good-quality chocolate this week but no real S.A.D. foods and was feeling 'pretty good considering it's January.' Her respiratory health was better (she was using her inhaler less than usual), she had lost some 'tummy fat', and she was feeling 'a lot more level than I normally would coming through Christmas.' Her good new habits had become ingrained and were now, she said, a part of her everyday life. 'I think it's pretty easy actually – because you stack it on, it's more achievable than cutting things out. I found it a lot easier than all the other diets I've tried. And if I can do a detox over Christmas, I can do anything.'

What next for Claire? She saw the Plan as being sustainable for her, long-term. 'The Stacking Plan has inspired me to take things forward. It really shows you how simple it is to eat and drink healthily – people don't do it though. If you can eat and drink sensibly and have a few treats then you don't feel deprived.'

Ollie found the final week easy, since he had stopped eating most junk food anyway – his only slip was a few biscuits on one day. He summed up his overall experience of the Plan thus:

'I really liked how the plan worked in introducing rules slowly – it feels a lot more sustainable with no horrible shocks for the body. You feel like you are making changes rather than sacrifices, and if I feel I have made a mistake on one rule I am still on it with the rest so psychologically it doesn't feel like a complete failure and it's easier to feel positive and get back on track. And as I started to feel the extra energy kicking in I was approaching the rules with the expectation that they would make me feel better.

'I eat a lot less stuff that makes me feel rubbish and when I have I know it, notice it and can correct it. When I feel my energy flagging I am more likely to give myself a boost with nutrition rather than sugar, refined carbs or coffee. The diet I now eat feels SO much healthier and energising. When I exercise I feel like I recover quicker and I generally feel a lot fitter and able to challenge myself more without it feeling damaging like it used to.

'My portion sizes are getting smaller, and I eat slower and more consciously, enjoy what I eat more than before and know better when I am full and it's time to stop eating. I have started to feel like I am losing weight faster since Christmas and because I feel that what I am eating now is sustainable I am pretty sure over the next few months I will continue to lose weight and get to a healthy BMI.

'I will continue with the plan as it just feels pretty normal to me now, not restrictive in any way. I feel OK that I can eat some stuff which is not so good every now and then and still stay on track. I feel like I have much more control over what I eat and how it makes me feel now.'

The Stacking Plan: what to do

So that's what to *eat*. This section describes what to *do* - four key lifestyle elements which are potent ingredients for health and happiness. These go hand-in-hand with healthful eating, with all five factors combining to create a powerful formula whose whole is greater than the sum of its parts. The four lifestyle elements are part of normal daily life in the Longevity Hot Spots, and up-to-date research shows that they are also highly beneficial to those of us living more modern lifestyles. Not doing them, on the other hand, can be positively detrimental.

If one or more of these elements is missing from your life or could be improved upon, you can use this section to think about how to address what is missing and find ways to incorporate it into your life. If this seems like a major overhaul, take it step by step, perhaps doing one small thing at a time and observing how much difference it makes. You are likely to find that the different activities described here leak into each other – when you start doing one, it leads to doing others, so that the pieces all end up slotting into each other like a very satisfying jigsaw.

The four elements are:

- Keep moving
- Relax
- Make the connection
- Have purpose

Keep moving

As a wise person once said: 'Exercise: you don't have time not to.' If you want to buy some extra healthy years, then one of the best investments you can make is to take regular exercise.

The dramatic effect on health of being physically active was observed after World War II when there was an epidemic of heart attacks in the UK. Researcher Jerry Morris set about finding out why, and he concluded that heart health and activity rates are strongly linked. Bus drivers in London, for example, who sat behind a wheel all day, were far more likely to die from a heart attack than bus conductors, who were constantly going up and down the stairs of double-decker buses.

Our bodies like to keep moving – if they don't, they start to malfunction and stagnate. Unfortunately, modern life can make constant movement quite difficult. To a large degree, chasing after wild game has been replaced by sitting at a desk sending emails, running around just for fun by watching TV, and climbing up trees to pick fruit by eating packets of crisps or biscuits. Modern 'couch potato syndrome' has serious repercussions for health: a study in *the Lancet* in 2012 concluded that lack of physical activity causes 5.3 million deaths per year, which makes having a sedentary lifestyle as dangerous as smoking (1).

If you are already physically active, then that is excellent. However, if you are fairly sedentary, then it may be time to think about ways to make physical movement a part of your day. This doesn't necessarily mean joining an expensive gym – walking around the block a couple of times a day, hula hooping whilst watching television, doing housework and going up and down the stairs are all ways of getting moving.

Combining healthy eating with exercise will greatly enhance the effects of both, which seems like common sense, but it has also been confirmed by a recent study (2). This same study also found that if inactivity were decreased by just ten per cent, it would prevent half a million deaths worldwide each year, which suggests that even a small change can make a big difference.

Exercise has the following good effects:

- It lowers blood pressure
- It lowers levels of homocysteine, a strong predictor of heart disease
- It lowers levels of 'bad' LDL cholesterol
- It improves muscle strength, including the heart muscle and muscles lining the colon
- It boosts circulation and lymphatic function
- It boosts white blood cell performance to enhance the immune system
- It lowers risk of cancers of the breast and colon
- It improves bone density so reducing the risk of osteoporosis
- It boosts metabolism and burns calories to aid weight loss
- It improves insulin sensitivity and balances blood glucose thus reducing the risk of diabetes and other chronic degenerative disease
- It improves mood by causing the release of endorphins and enhances cognitive function by stimulating blood flow to the brain and growth factors which enable neuronal cells to grow
- It stimulates anti-ageing growth hormone
- It reduces levels of the 'stress' hormone, cortisol

How much is enough?

Most experts recommend that we exercise for around half an hour to an hour three or more days a week as a basic minimum. However, if you can't fit that into your day, even ten minutes a day of brisk walking has been shown to cut heart attack risk and benefit health (3). James Levine MD, author of *Get Up! Why Your Chair Is Killing You and What You Can Do About It* (2014), cites a study showing that if people in the US walked for just eighteen minutes extra daily there would be a thirteen per cent reduction in premature deaths, which would rank alongside the greatest health advances in modern history. Other recent studies have shown that when older people do very short bursts of intensive exercise for just a few seconds, they have significant improvements in health – which also means that it's never too late to start (4).

Beware of over-exercising, since doing too much intensive exercise raises levels of ageing free radicals, lowers immunity, and promotes the pro-ageing stress hormone, cortisol. A recent study of 18-year-old males training to join the Israel Defence Force showed that over-exercising is also likely to cause a low blood count, and it is well-established that athletes often have poor immunity (5).

Aerobic exercise which makes you get out of breath is best for the heart, since it gets the heart pumping and helps make the lungs strong. It also boosts circulation, getting the nutrients around the bloodstream to where they are needed and sending lurking toxins on their way.

Do it outdoors

Taking exercise out of doors is especially good for us because being in sunlight allows the body to make a very important nutrient – vitamin D. Vitamin D, also known as 'the sunshine vitamin', is manufactured in the body when the skin is exposed to ultraviolet rays, and it is essential for good health. It is found in small amounts in some foods, such as fish, cheese, and egg yolks, but sunlight is the most reliable source.

Vitamin D deficiency is a serious problem in the modern world, sometimes referred to as an 'unseen epidemic' which is estimated to affect up to forty per cent of the US female population, twenty five per cent of British people and a billion

Europeans. Lack of vitamin D is linked with health problems including cancer, heart disease, diabetes, arthritis, multiple sclerosis and osteoporosis (6).

Those of us who live in higher latitudes where sunshine levels are low need to spend ten to twenty minutes outside every day during warmer months, or, if that isn't possible, an hour each day at weekends and on holidays, in order to make enough vitamin D for our needs (7). Dark-skinned people require more sunlight than pale-skinned people in order to get enough vitamin D and should take extra care to get outside regularly. Those who live in sunnier climates, especially if pale-skinned, will need less sun exposure time than those in colder areas.

What about skin cancer? Obviously we don't want to be over-exposed to bright sunshine, but nor do we want to be deficient in vitamin D. Vitamin D may also help protect us from skin cancer, since it protects us from precancerous changes to skin cells when they are exposed to UVB rays. However, we can only manufacture vitamin D when we do not use a sunscreen with a factor of above eight (8). Since the latest research suggests that using sunscreen even with factor fifty does not prevent skin cancer, this suggests that going out in mild sunshine or at least daylight without sunscreen may be ideal (9). Either way, burning or excessive exposure to sunlight should always be avoided and if you have very pale skin or concerns about skin cancer take extra care to avoid harsh sunlight.

Exercise ideas

Here are some ideas for exercise and movement – choose one or more activities you enjoy and can realistically fit into your day. Don't forget to warm up before starting any vigorous exercise and to cool down afterwards by slowing down and doing stretches.

- Brisk walking (or using a treadmill or treadmill desk

whilst working)
- Bicycling (or using an exercise bike)
- Dancing (eg belly dancing, Zumba, tango, salsa, capoeira)
- Martial Arts (eg taekwondo, kung fu, karate, kickboxing)
- Yoga
- Pilates
- Swimming
- Sports such as golf, tennis, football, rugby, or hockey
- Aerobics and fitness classes
- Rowing (canoes, boats or kayaks)
- Hula hooping
- Doing housework and/or gardening
- Walking up and down the stairs
- Using a balance ball

Relax

Tension is who you think you should be.
Relaxation is who you are.
Chinese proverb

Address your stress

Most of us who live a modern lifestyle are rarely short of stressful events in our daily lives. Whether it's meeting the bills, being stuck in traffic, the children, death, marriage, not being married, divorce, deadlines, or something else – there's always something waiting to get our cortisol flowing, our blood pressure rising, and our nerves fraying.

Stress was fine back in the day when it was caused by, for example, someone or something trying to eat or kill us and we needed extra adrenaline or cortisol in order to deal with the situation. Those 'fight-or-flight' type hormones were useful so that we could run away fast or have the presence of mind to hit our enemy over the head with a club.

Of course, today, we sometimes have to deal with parallel situations, such as setting the frying pan on fire, or being yelled at by an enraged driver who seems to think that their bad driving is our fault. However, on top of these *acute* stressors, we also tend to have a lot of *chronic* stressors – more general life circumstances which may cause us long-term, low-level stress, such as work or relationship issues. Instead of using our stress hormones usefully and in a short burst, we stew in their toxic juices, as it were.

This is why stress is strongly linked with chronic diseases such as heart disease, diabetes, and depression. The stress hormone, cortisol, which becomes chronically raised with chronic stress, lowers immunity, accelerates bone loss, disrupts blood sugar levels, and is toxic to the brain (1). Stress also triggers the production of ageing free radicals and causes the release of acidic phosphorus into the bloodstream. In short, stress speeds up the ageing process.

Many of us have genuine, unavoidable stressors to deal with, but to a certain extent we can control the degree to which we get stressed by those stressors. One of the things that researchers have noticed about long-lived people, including those in Longevity Hot Spots, is that they tend to have good resilience to any stressors they are presented with: one study of centenarians, for example, found that people who live long tend to have 'stress-resistant personalities.' (2).

If you feel that you don't have time to relax, remember that taking just a bit of time out to do so can buy you extra quality years in the end. Here are some ideas about how to address your stress:

Look after your adrenals

If you feel 'tired but wired' much of the time, struggle to get out of bed in the mornings, have a 'second wind' in the evening, have difficulties coping with day-to-day life, can be irritable for no apparent reason, need stimulants such as coffee and sugar to keep you awake, sleep badly, perhaps crave salty foods, and possibly suffer from lethargy and depression, you may well have 'adrenal fatigue'. Adrenal fatigue simply means that your adrenal glands, which have to work overtime when you are stressed, are functioning below par. It is very common for people to have adrenal fatigue as a result of long-term chronic stress, burning the candle at both ends, and/or not eating the right things.

The adrenals can be restored effectively by improving the diet, taking certain supplements, and taking time out to rest, relax, and take exercise. I often see people in my clinic who have some degree of adrenal fatigue and who respond very well to these measures. Two excellent natural treatments for adrenal fatigue are Siberian Ginseng and ashwagandha – please consult a professional who has knowledge of these before taking them. There are also some excellent supplements for adrenal fatigue on the market – again, please consult a qualified practitioner.

Meditate

Meditation is an effective way to reduce stress which improves well-being so much that it is used in some hospitals to aid the healing process and reduce pain. Transcendental meditation in particular is deeply relaxing and has been found to be especially effective at turning back the biological clock, enhancing the body's self-repair systems, and reducing biomarkers of ageing such as lowering blood pressure, improving insulin sensitivity and improving cardiac health, all of which can be linked with stress (3). One study of transcendental meditation indicated that those who practised it had fifty five per cent fewer hospital admissions for cancer and eighty seven per cent fewer admissions for heart disease than non-meditators (4).

There are many different types of meditation including transcendental meditation, compassionate meditation, mindfulness, breath-watching, and empty mind meditation. There are any number of books and classes on the subject, so if you are interested you should be able to find something to suit you. In the meantime, when you feel stressed, simply sit still for a few minutes and keep your attention on your breath, whilst allowing your thoughts to float past.

Simple 10-step meditation technique

1. Find a quiet place to sit for 30-40 minutes.
2. Sit cross-legged on the floor or against the wall in a way that enables you to be comfortable for the duration of meditation.
3. Keep your back straight and your neck aligned with your spine, with your head tilted slightly forward.
4. Keep perfectly still.
5. Half-close your eyes – this will help prevent both

161

daydreams and visible objects from distracting you.

6. Relax your shoulders.
7. Slightly constrict your sphincter so as to preserve internal energy circulation.
8. Exhale the old air from your lungs with a few breaths, then take a few deep breaths. Start to breathe normally, with smooth soft breaths, and focus on your breath.
9. Focus on internal sounds and ignore external sounds.
10. Stray thoughts will start to come. Let them pass through. Do not focus on them but do not try to push them away either. Simply let your internal dialogue become weaker and weaker, and do nothing. Keep focussing on your breathing only.

Deep breathing exercises

Deep breathing enables oxygenation of body tissues and has a relaxing, rejuvenating effect. Stress has the opposite effect, causing us to breathe more shallowly. Note that whilst healthy cells thrive in a highly oxygenated environment, cancer cells do not. Low oxygen levels also create acidic conditions in the body.

Try this simple deep breathing method:

1. Sit cross-legged in loose clothes and keep your spine straight. Relax.
2. Inhale and exhale slowly, expanding your chest and lower abdomen as you breathe in. Count to five.
3. Breathe out all the old stale air and imagine the fresh, new air coming in and reaching to all the parts of your body.
4. Remember not to overdo it, as this may lead to hyper-oxygenation which can cause dizziness. Do what feels natural.

Meditation, aerobic exercise and yoga are all also ways to improve deep breathing, and getting out to a park or the countryside whenever you can is another good way to oxygenate yourself.

Put your head in your hands

We are all familiar with the classic image of someone putting their head in their hands hopelessly or clapping their hand to their head when given bad news. In fact, there are some real benefits to adopting this despairing position.

According to the practice of kinesiology, there are areas on the forehead called 'neurovascular reflex points' – the two slightly bumpy areas of bone situated halfway between the eyebrows and the hairline. Putting your hand here helps release stress and encourages blood flow to the front of the brain where it is needed for clear thought during a crisis.

Children are reported to find this technique helpful when struggling with homework, and it is also a handy technique to use *before* you enter a potentially stressful situation.

Get plenty of sleep

Not getting enough sleep can make us 'tired but wired', especially if we start relying too much on caffeine. Sleep problems are very common, with around one in three Britons thought to get insufficient sleep and between 50 and 70 million Americans being reported to suffer from sleep disorders.

Sleep not only helps to reduce stress but it is also important for keeping your immune system strong, allowing the nervous system and organs to rest and repair, keeping glucose levels on the straight and narrow, and releasing those all-important hormones which tell our bodies what to do. Lack of sleep is associated with increased risk of chronic disease such as heart disease, obesity and diabetes (5). Edward L. Schneider, of the Leonard Davis School of Gerontology, UCLA, has said 'To age successfully, you must get a good night's sleep.'

Experts differ on how much sleep we need, but it seems that between seven and eight hours is about the right amount, although it varies between individuals and age groups. Teens need between eight and a half and nine and a half hours each night, and older people tend to sleep less.

In order to get a good night's sleep try the following:

1. Go to bed at roughly the same time every night and get up at the same time every morning, since hormone production depends on a 24-hour clock and sleep hormones will work better this way.
2. Avoid caffeine or sugar in the evening and keep alcohol to a minimum or avoid it completely, since although it can make you feel sleepy at first, the sugar will have a stimulating effect later.
3. Avoid eating a large meal too close to bed time, and avoid going to bed hungry. A warm milky drink has been found in studies to promote sleep – I don't recommend cows' milk, but oat milk or soy milk are useful alternatives.
4. Make sure you eat plenty of green leafy vegetables as these contain magnesium, the 'calming' mineral, which helps promote sleep. If you get leg cramps or regularly wake in the early hours this can indicate magnesium deficiency and you may benefit from taking a magnesium supplement.
5. Try eating carbohydrates, including plenty of vegetables but also some starchy carbohydrates, at the evening meal, as this promotes the production of serotonin which aids sleep. Bananas and turkey, which contain tryptophan which is a precursor to serotonin, can also help. Cheese also contains tryptophan, and one study conducted in the UK in 2005 indicated that eating cheese before bed seems to promote good sleep as well as pleasant dreams, including dreams about the film star Johnny Depp. (However, cheese has many health drawbacks, and it comes as no surprise to find that this study was conducted by the British Cheese Board).

6. Avoid watching television or looking at a computer screen before bed, as the light from electronic devices is stimulating and interferes with the sleep-promoting hormone, melatonin.

7. Keep lights dim and when you turn out the light make sure the bedroom is fully dark so as to boost melatonin production.

8. Have a bedtime ritual to relax you, such as having a bath and then reading a book.

9. If you tend to lie in bed worrying about the next day, try making a list of everything you have to do and putting it aside. Then, once in bed, think of eight things which happened that day which made you feel happy. These don't have to be major events – enjoying a nice cup of tea or seeing a pretty flower is enough. Doing this will stimulate the production of dopamine which promotes sleep.

10. Try relaxing your body part by part, starting at the toes and working your way up to your head and arms, when you turn out the light. You can also listen to a relaxation CD to help you do this.

11. If you think you may have adrenal fatigue (see above), addressing this should help you to sleep better.

12. If household sounds, such as noisy pipes, a snoring partner, or the road outside keep you awake, try using ear plugs at night. This simple measure can make all the difference to your quality of sleep. Eye masks are also useful for blocking out light. An eye mask and ear plugs may not be the most romantic look, but at least it can help you to be less grumpy in the morning.

Have a good laugh

Laughter is a great stress reducer which relaxes us, reduces levels of the stress hormone cortisol, lowers blood pressure, boosts immunity and triggers the release of endorphins which reduce pain and give us a sense of well-being. It also gives the heart, diaphragm, and abdominal muscles a good workout.

In the 1960s, the American journalist Norman Cousins was diagnosed with ankylosing spondylitis and was told that he was very unlikely ever to recover. He was sent to hospital where he was given thirty-eight painkillers daily. Cousins decided the only way ahead was to take an active role in his own recovery, so he discharged himself and set about devising what came to be known as his 'laughter cure'. Every day, Cousins watched Marx Brothers films and had his nurse read amusing books to him, and made sure to have a good ten-minute belly laugh at least once a day. He also nurtured a sense of love, faith, hope and a positive attitude and took huge doses of vitamin C. Within a relatively short space of time, Cousins had recovered enough from his illness to return to work full time.

In order to induce laughter, try watching a funny video, reading a funny book, or just laughing for no reason. 'Laughter yoga', which originated in Mumbai in India, is an activity in which people meet in a park, raise their arms in the air, and laugh repeatedly until their laughter becomes real and contagious; weight loss and dramatically-reduced depression are just two of the reported benefits. 'Laughter clubs' are popular in the UK and the US today so there may well be one near you.

Have a good cry

If you sometimes don't know whether to laugh or cry, that's fine, because crying can also be helpful when it comes to relieving stress and finding ways to relax. If you are bottling something up, having a good cathartic cry can help relieve the pressure. To 'express' means literally to 'squeeze out' – so it makes sense to 'express' any bottled-up tension or unhappiness.

Crying also helps deliver oxygen to cells and triggers the release of relaxing brain chemicals and endorphins. And, according to US biochemist and 'tear expert' Dr William Frey, tears can help remove toxins from the body and reduce levels of chemicals which build up in the body during times of stress.

If you aren't one for crying, but think it might do you good to squeeze some tears out, try helping them along by putting on a poignant piece of music or watching a sad film – whatever works for you. Don't rely on chopping onions, since Frey's research shows that only tears triggered by a sad movie, rather than onion-chopping, do the trick.

An alternative to crying is to express anger, without hurting anyone obviously. It can help just to say 'I am angry because…', if you can achieve that without shouting or hitting. It has often been noted that Mediterranean men are good at *expressing* (letting out) their feelings, rather than letting them simmer unhealthily. The ultra-healthy, long-lived Sardinians are known for speaking their minds when feeling displeasure – hence the word *sardonic*, which comes from the island. This ability to express feelings may well be a factor in keeping blood pressure down.

Eat chocolate

The image of a tear-stained girl eating chocolates in bed may be a cliché but it's true – chocolate can make you feel better and reduce stress.

Chocolate triggers the release of pleasure-inducing endorphins and contains a range of feel-good substances including tryptophan, magnesium and theobromine. A 2009 study showed that eating one bar of chocolate each day for two weeks reduced stress hormones; whilst in a 2004 study entitled 'sweet babies', women who ate chocolate regularly during pregnancy reported not only lower levels of stress, but happier babies (6).

If you are going to eat chocolate, though, don't overdo it, as most chocolate contains sugar. Pure cacao is probably the best option, since it is a purely natural product without any sugar. Alternatively, go for good quality organic dark chocolate with as little sugar as possible.

Take regular exercise

Getting regular exercise is also an excellent way to keep stress at bay. It lowers levels of the stress hormone cortisol, it triggers the release of feel-good endorphins, and it reduces anxiety and depression (7). Taking exercise also helps us use glucose and insulin more effectively, so helping balance blood sugar levels, which should help with sleep quality. Getting physically tired should also, of course, aid sleep.

Different types of exercise may suit different moods or personalities. Going for a walk or a run in a place of natural beauty, rather than using the treadmill at the gym surrounded by people in lycra with perfect bodies, may be particularly enjoyable and therefore de-stressing for some. Hitting a punch bag may be a good way to release pent-up frustration, whilst yoga promotes calm and relaxation. Dance classes involving music you enjoy are excellent for triggering endorphin production as well as socialising with others.

Make the connections

Count your age with friends, but not with years.
Anon.

An epidemic of loneliness

Loneliness has become increasingly common in the UK and the US during the last few decades. According to surveys, almost one third of people in the UK and the US now lives in a single-person household, one in ten people do not have a single close friend, and almost a fifth who took part in one survey said that in the previous two weeks they rarely or never felt loved (1, 2). One report pointed out that this is despite the fact that most people are surrounded by others in their daily life.

Loneliness can affect people of all ages: research has shown that members of the age 18-34 age group are most likely to feel lonely 'often', whilst a third of over-75s spend twelve hours a day alone, with one in ten over-75s reported to feel 'intensely lonely all of the time' (3, 4). And according to Esther Rantzen of the charity Childline, children, like adults, are facing an 'epidemic of loneliness', as a result of the decline in family life (5).

Loneliness does not necessarily mean just being alone for a period of time, but is as much to do with feeling chronically isolated from others through lack of meaningful contact. We can be surrounded by others and still feel disconnected, just as we can enjoy episodes of solitude. In traditional societies such as those in the Longevity Hot Spots, people may have periods of time alone but they are also part of a community of extended family, neighbours and friends, and they are likely to work and socialise with others in a way that gives them a sense of belonging. In our modern world, by contrast, there is less likely to be a ready-made community around people in which to have meaningful interactions or to have a well-defined role.

Loneliness and health

Loneliness, apart from being unpleasant, also has major implications for our physical health. Loneliness has actually been found to be more damaging to health than obesity and as bad as smoking fifteen cigarettes per day; research also suggests that lonely people are fifty per cent more likely to die over a seven-and-a-half-year period than others (6, 7).

According to loneliness expert John Capiocco, co-author of *Loneliness: Human Nature and Our Need for Social Connection* (2009), loneliness causes lower immunity, higher levels of stress hormones, damage to cardiovascular function, inflammation, and is disruptive to cellular function on a deeper level, which causes faster ageing. Lonely adults also tend to drink more alcohol, sleep less well, and to get less exercise.

Connecting with others, on the other hand, helps make us healthy and happy. Here are some of the ways in which that happens, and some tips for forging connections.

Friends with health benefits

Good friends help us to have good health, according to numerous studies. Being with people we like increases levels of the 'pleasure' brain chemicals such as serotonin and endorphins and helps keep blood pressure down. Being with friends also causes us to release oxytocin, the 'cuddle hormone' which has numerous health benefits (see below for more on oxytocin). One study showed that older people with good friendship networks outlived others by twenty two per cent (8).

In our urban societies it can be easy to lose touch with other people, despite the fact that there are thousands or millions of them living nearby. If you feel that your social life could do with some improving, there may be some proactive measures you can take. Making more effort to get together

170

with friends, taking the dog for a walk and chatting to other walkers, working at an internet café instead of alone at home, and joining sports or dance classes are all obvious way to get out and meet people with whom you may find you have something in common.

There are also many groups which have been set up to help bring people together. These include groups such as:

- MeetUp – this is a way to find other people in your area who share interests with you and includes a wide range of activities. See www.meetup.com
- Netmums – this provides an online forum as well as actual contact, with 10,000 mums getting together every month via the 'meet a mum' scheme. See www.netmums.com
- Silver Line (set up by Child Line's founder, Esther Rantzen), which provides 'information, friendship and advice' for older people. See www.thesilverline.org.uk
- Men in Sheds – this is run by Age UK and is designed for older men to get together to do activities such as woodwork, skills sharing and socialising – check the Age UK website for details of a group near you. See www. ageuk.org.uk
- Participle – this is a movement which aims to address social issues such as family problems, employment for older people, and wellness. See http://participle.net
- Dating sites – there are, of course, numerous dating sites and friendship sites which enable people to connect over the internet and meet up in real life.

Give in order to receive

We've all heard the saying 'giving is receiving.' It turns out that this ancient piece of advice is rooted in biochemical fact. Giving to others can create a sense of belonging and reciprocity which brings blood pressure down, boosts endorphin levels, and strengthens immunity, all of which contribute to long life and wellbeing.

Both giving and receiving are likely to be beneficial, but it seems that giving comes out tops. In one study, it was found that stress caused thirty per cent higher mortality in those who did not help others, but no increase for those who did (9). And in a five-year study of older people, those who were helpful to others had a sixty per cent lower chance of dying during the study period than others. This effect was put down to factors such as creating motivation to stay alive, providing a sense of empowerment, and reducing loneliness. Being on the receiving end, however, made no measurable difference (10).

In the Longevity Hot Spots, centenarians in Bama have told longevity researchers that 'doing good deeds' keeps them healthy, whilst Okinawans value the concept of giving and reciprocity very highly and have their own word for it, *yuuimaru*.

If you would like to do something to help others but do not have any friends, relatives or neighbours who you know of who could use your support, there are organisations such as Volunteer England which can help. See www.volunteering. org.uk to find a group near you.

Marry...

Being married can have either a beneficial or a detrimental effect on health, depending on how well any given couple gets on. A UK study showed that married people, especially men, live up to three years longer than unmarried people (11). This particular study did not find the same results for co-habiting couples, but other studies suggest that having a partner or a spouse can be good for us (12). And sex three times weekly between long-term partners makes them look up to ten years younger because of anti-ageing hormones produced as a result, according to Dr David Weeks, author of *Secrets of the Superyoung* (1998). However, sex three times weekly outside of a stable relationship was found to be ageing.

Marriage is unlikely to boost health if the couple does not

get on, however. In one study, couples were asked to discuss a marital issue they wished to change, and gave them a small blister on the arm. The blister healed more quickly when the discussion between the couple was harmonious than if they were nasty and sarcastic to each other (13).

…or get a dog, or eat chilli and chocolate

One of the reasons why having a spouse or partner is good for us is thanks to the effects of the 'cuddle hormone', oxytocin, which is produced when we interact lovingly not just with spouses but with other people generally as well as with pets.

Oxytocin is anti-inflammatory and it helps lower blood pressure, helps combat obesity and diabetes, promotes wound-healing, lowers levels of ageing cortisol and increases production of anti-ageing growth hormone (14).

In Japanese study entitled 'Pet Dogs Rival Humans for Emotional Satisfaction', it was found that interacting with a pet dog boosts the production of oxytocin; presumably the same would go for spending quality time with a cat, but these particular researchers happen to be dog-lovers (15).

Hugging friends, relatives and romantic partners also increases oxytocin levels, as do singing, reading, looking at paintings you like, listening to music, eating chocolate, and consuming capsaicin from chilli peppers.

Change your perceptions with cognitive behavioural therapy

Loneliness expert John Capiocco believes that loneliness is often a subjective experience, and is more to do with the way people perceive themselves in a social situation than the amount of social contact with others they have. He claims that the most effective ways to reduce loneliness and feel connected use cognitive behavioural therapy techniques to shift the way people perceive social situations they find themselves in, rather than simply increasing the amount of social contact. Cognitive behavioural therapy (CBT) is available on the NHS – to find out if you qualify for CBT you need to see your GP and ask for a referral.

Have purpose

We all need a reason to get out of bed every morning – a *raison d'etre*, a *plana de vida*, a purpose in life. Having a sense of meaning and purpose keeps us going, whilst not having one can drag down both our mental and physical health.

In a recent study of 1,238 elderly people in Chicago, it was found that those who had a strong sense of purpose were about half as likely to die over the follow-up period than those with a poor sense of purpose, even after other factors were accounted for (1). Another study of over 6,000 people showed that those who claimed to have a sense of purpose at the start of the fourteen-year study period tended to outlive those who did not, no matter what age they were when they found direction and purpose, and no matter what it was that they felt purposeful about (2).

Why might this be? It could be that purposeful people have healthier lifestyles or that healthier people are more purposeful. One study also suggests that having a sense of purpose directly reduces stress levels. In this study, students were asked to take train journeys in which the other passengers were from different races, with the intention of raising the students' stress levels, since being with other races is a known stressor. Those students who were given tasks to make them focus on their purpose in life during the journey did not experience an increase in stress, whereas the others did (3). Since increased stress raises blood pressure, this suggests that having a sense of purpose could be beneficial for heart health. In another study of older people it was found that those who are more optimistic have 73 per cent lower rates of heart failure than those who are pessimistic, which could be because being positive also lowers blood pressure (4).

There may also be other factors at work. One intriguing study revealed that people with purpose are less likely to have cognitive symptoms of Alzheimer's Disease than others even when they have the characteristic plaques and tangles in their brains which characterise the illness. On average, the rate of cognitive decline was 30 per cent lower in those who felt a sense of purpose (5).

Having a sense of purpose seems to have other beneficial physical effects, too. In an ongoing US programme named 'Experience Corps', over-55s are paired up with kindergarten children to help with literacy. Originally the aim was to improve literacy in the children, but there has been another, unexpected result – the physical mobility, stamina and flexibility of the older people involved is found to improve, and levels of depression drop. This finding has been put down to a renewed sense of purpose in the over-55s having some kind of physical effect on the body.

So: how do we go about living our life with purpose? Here are some tips.

Set realistic goals

You may have some major life goals which you could more proactively pursue in order to have a sense of direction. If so, try working out a strategy for how to achieve these, making sure to keep your goals realistic, or at least within the realms of possibility. The sky may be the limit, or you may need to take smaller steps for now.

If you feel that your life lacks purpose in some way but you are not sure where you are going, you may need to reassess what you do or who you are doing it for. A dead-end job for an ungrateful boss, relentless child-rearing without help, not knowing what your strengths are, not having enough to do… these can all lead to a sense of purposelessness. Try sitting down and asking yourself what will make you feel glad to get up in the morning, and make an effort to incorporate those things in your life. Sometimes it only takes something small to effect a big change.

Take up a hobby

Doing things we really enjoy can help us feel a sense of purpose as we become absorbed and, after doing the activity, feel a sense of achievement and satisfaction. Learning a musical instrument, doing an art or sculpture class, weeding the garden, doing voluntary work, walking the dog, swimming, doing embroidery, playing chess, joining a book club or doing dance classes are just some examples of a great many activities available which can give us a sense of meaning and purpose.

Taking up a hobby may be particularly valuable after retirement. The year after retirement is known to be a vulnerable time for older people, who can lose their sense of purpose, which in turn is bad for health - a study by Shell Oil found that those who retired at the age of fifty five were more likely to die than those who retired at sixty five (6). In the Longevity Hot Spots I have visited, there is no such thing as retirement, and old people feel needed and are kept busy, which must be one reason for their typical sprightliness.

Turn lemons into lemonade

Whilst life CAN be unfair, we have a lot of power to decide for ourselves how to perceive the events in our lives. What for some people might be a cruel blow, for others can be an interesting challenge. Whilst life happens to some, passively suffering the hand they are dealt, others choose for themselves the course they will take, and if something goes wrong, they simply learn from that lesson and take another course.

'Purposeful living' includes the ability to derive meaning from life experiences, both every-day and extraordinary ones, and to be focussed and intentional in our thoughts and actions. Andrew Zolli, author of *Resilience: Why Things Bounce Back*, writes that people with purpose can 'cognitively reappraise situations and regulate emotions, turning life's proverbial lemons into lemonade.'

The practice of hypnotherapy teaches that our brains do

not know the difference between thoughts and reality, which means that we can react emotionally to a thought even if we know that thought to be untrue. We can therefore override negative or victim-like emotional states and train our brains to see things positively with a bit of practice. Hypnotherapy as well as Cognitive Behavioural Therapy (CBT) can be particularly useful in learning how to undo negative thinking and live with more purposefulness and positivity. This in turn can have a positive effect on our physical wellbeing, since our physical wellbeing is strongly linked with our mental wellbeing.

Meditation and the dung ball

Studies suggest that meditating can help maintain the length of our telomeres, which in turn is linked with longer life, and that one of the effects of meditation is that it gives us a sense of purpose (7). According to Victor Strecher, professor of health behaviour in the US and author of the book and app *On Purpose*, this sense of purpose we get from meditating is itself directly linked with the effect on telomeres. Strecher's book is inspired by the loss of his 19-year-old daughter, and is about a dung beetle whose purpose in life is to push a faecal ball around. 'If you think about dung beetles', he says, 'they push this giant ball of shit up to 100 yards in a perfectly straight line; it's the most purposeful thing you'll ever see in your life' (8).

If you wish to take up meditation as a way of feeling a sense of purpose, there is more about how to meditate in the chapter 'Relax…', and a quick look on the internet should help you find books to read or courses near you.

Have faith

Having some form of spiritual faith gives people a sense of deeper meaning and purposefulness in life, as well as making people feel connected both with other worshippers and with a higher power. Studies show that people who practise a religion live longer; one reason could be the sense of purpose which having faith provides. In all of the Longevity Hot Spots, spirituality of some kind is an important part of everyday life.

Surround yourself with people you like

As we saw in 'Make the Connections', being with people whose company we enjoy is good for our physical and mental health. Surrounding ourselves with people we are fond of or find interesting can also help provide a sense of purpose by reassuring us of our own identity, inspiring us to do the same types of things as they do and being there to talk to if we feel we have lost our way or need a few pointers.

Some other suggestions for having a sense of purpose:

Create a daily routine, as flexible as you wish it to be, to give your day structure and a sense of direction.

- Go for a walk to clear your head – this can be an amazingly effective way to find solutions to problems and give you a renewed sense of direction.
- Do not compare your life with others, but focus on what YOU are doing instead.
- Give some thought to why you do the things you do and make sure you have good reasons for doing them.

Recipes

The subject of *what to actually eat* is a big one for most of my clients who are trying to improve their diets. My advice is to make sure you stick to the basic principles and you can't go far wrong. Make sure you use plenty of fruit and vegetables, the right proteins, carbohydrates and fats, and minimal processed or refined foods. And, this may sound a bit ridiculous, but it's true: don't forget to go shopping, because it's not easy to make a meal when you don't have any ingredients to make it with.

I like simple recipes, probably because I have to cook so many meals for my children (surely over 10,000 by now) and I don't often make anything elaborate as I tend to be a bit last-minute. I just make sure to have lots of vegetables in the fridge, a full fruit bowl, a protein always ready, and some staples on the shelves, and that way there is always a nutritious and satisfying meal to be thrown together. I have included some recipes here which are a mix of standard recipes I have come across, recipes I have found in the Longevity Hot Spots, and what I have invented at home.

There are also endless Stacking Plan-friendly recipes on the internet, in cook books, and which you can invent for yourself. If you love cooking, fantastic – you are bound to come up with some wonderful creations. Try looking for high-vegetable recipes, Paleo recipes, Asian recipes, Mediterranean recipes, and wheat-free and dairy-free recipes for inspiration. At first it may take some conscious effort to eat well, but after a while it will become habit and you won't have to think about it much.

If you eat out often, try to choose places where you can stick to the principles as far as you can – ones which serve plenty of vegetables and fish, for example. If you have lunch at the office and there is nothing suitable to eat nearby you may find it best to make your own lunch and take it with you, and I have included several salads which you may find useful for that purpose.

I haven't included any cake or pudding recipes in this section because there are so many fantastic recipes out there for less-sinful sweet treats such as raw cakes, gluten-free baking and even Paleo-style baking, and I tend not to do a lot of baking myself.

Shopping list

Here is a list of items you will find useful to keep at home so that you can rustle up healthful recipes at short notice:
- A variety of fresh vegetables and root vegetables
- Frozen vegetables (peas and spinach are my favourites)
- Fermented vegetables such as sauerkraut and kimchi
- Fresh fish, chicken or lean meat
- Soy products such as tofu, miso, tempeh, tamari soya sauce
- Organic free-range eggs
- Yoghurt and/or soya yoghurt
- A variety of fresh fruit
- Dried beans and lentils
- Nuts and seeds
- Ground almonds
- Desiccated coconut
- Nut butters
- Wheat-free flours; gluten-free flours
- Porridge flakes (eg oat flakes, buckwheat flakes, quinoa flakes, millet flakes)
- Wheat-free pastas and noodles
- Maple syrup
- Honey
- All-fruit jam
- Coconut oil, extra-virgin olive oil, and avocado oil or groundnut oil
- Ghee and/or organic butter
- Good-quality sea salt or Himalayan salt

- Fresh pepper for grinding
- Dried mixed herbs and fresh herbs
- Herb teas
- Green tea
- Coffee substitute
- Non-dairy milks such as oat milk, rice milk, nut milk and soya milk

Removing anti-nutrients from legumes, grains, pseudograins, nuts, and seeds

As you know from the Proteins and Carbohydrates weeks, legumes (beans and peas), whole grains, pseudograins and nuts and seeds contain certain *anti-nutrients*.

The subject of removing anti-nutrients is a big one, and it is beyond the scope of this book to cover it in full. I have outlined some basic methods below, but if you wish to find out more, there are dozens of websites devoted to the subject. Here are a few useful ones I have found:

http://www.westonaprice.org/health-topics/living-with-phytic-acid/

http://thepaleodiet.com/beans-and-legumes-are-they-paleo/

http://nourishedkitchen.com/soaking-grains-nuts-legumes/

http://www.livestrong.com/article/527681-how-to-ferment-whole-grains/

Soaking

Soaking beans, grains, pseudograins, or their flours in water causes the release of an enzyme called phytase which breaks down varying amounts of phytates, depending on the food in question. Warm water at a temperature of 60 C is best for beans as it has been found to reduce as much phytate content after three hours' soaking as cold water removes in eighteen hours. A hot plate on a low setting or a reptile basking light (if you happen to have one of these) are recommended ways of keeping the temperature warm.

Grains may also benefit from warm water, but the research has yet to be done so I cannot advise on soaking times but they may be shorter than for cold water for some grains.

Soaking has the additional benefit of removing oligosaccharides from beans, which can cause gas, and if you see foam on the water, that's the soapy saponins coming out. Remove the water after soaking your beans or grains and rinse, then use fresh water to cook.

Tinned beans have not been soaked and are lower in nutrients due to canning methods, so are not a solution to the problem of phytates in beans. If you do find you need to use a tin of beans for an emergency thrown-together meal, when you open the tin you will probably see foam from saponins, so give them a good rinse.

Soaking times:

Legumes (eg beans, lentils): 12-18 hours, ideally in warm water

Wheat, rye flour: 12-24 hours

Buckwheat, millet (grains or flakes): approx 7 hours

Quinoa (grains): 12-24 hours

Quinoa (flakes): approx. 7-8 hours

Brown rice, oats: 7 hours in cold water with buckwheat (this works best since they contain very little phytase of their own).

Soaking in acidic water

Soaking beans, grains, pseudograins or their flours in water which is slightly acidic triggers the release of phytase. Use one teaspoon of lemon or apple cider vinegar per cup of water; you can also use a cultured milk product such as kefir or buttermilk. However, many cooks prefer soaking in water without acid as they find that herbs and other flavours permeate the beans better when acid is not used.

Cooking

Cooking helps remove protease inhibitors but reduces only a negligible amount of phytates. Cooking in bone broth is a good idea since this causes the release of calcium from the bones which can offset some of the mineral-robbing effects of phytates.

Cooking reduces lectins, whilst pressure-cooking is thought to eliminate them completely.

Activating nuts and seeds

Nuts and seeds are often high in phytates; soaking and dehydrating ('activating') them will remove some of these. The basic method is to soak the nuts or seeds in warm water for several hours and then dehydrate them in a dehydrator or low oven for several hours. This may sound like a hassle, but it is actually very easy and it makes the nuts deliciously light and crunchy – it works particularly well for almonds – as well as more nutritious.

Activation can take up to 24 hours, so for individual nut-activating times you will need to consult one of the many internet sites covering this subject (I recently read one with the comment underneath: 'do I have to take the chocolate coating off first?'). Alternatively, you can buy activated nuts and seeds at some health food shops, if you can get past the price tag.

Blanched almonds and almond flour do not need to be activated, because the phytates are mainly contained in the outer skin.

Roasting and dry-frying nuts and seeds

You can soak nuts and seeds then roast or dry-fry them if you do not want to dehydrate them, but avoid cooking them on a high heat or for too long as this may damage their omega 6 essential fats. It is possible that heating nuts and seeds without soaking them also makes them more digestible, although more research is needed – my daughter gets a stomach ache if she eats raw seeds, but if I fry them in a little tamari soya sauce on a low heat for a minute or two she doesn't.

Sprouting

Sprouting reduces phytate content (up to around 50 or 60 %, depending on the food in question); for best results soak and then sprout. Sprouting should always be undertaken with caution as it can encourage the growth of *e. coli* – check the origin of the food you are sprouting with the retailer and make sure that you sprout in hygienic conditions.

You can sprout wheat or rye to make sprouted bread, or you can buy it ready-made – this is a moist, filling, nutrient-dense bread which also has lower levels of gluten than ordinary bread.

Fermenting (grains, pseudograins)

Fermenting grains, pseudograins and flours with the use of a yoghurt culture is thought to reduce some of the phytate content as well as the gluten content of gluten-containing grains. Fermenting also triggers the production of enzymes which increase the nutrient content of the food.

I sometimes ferment porridge flakes and flours by putting them in a bowl and adding a little warm water and a couple of tablespoonsful of live plain yoghurt or soy yoghurt. I leave it overnight in a warm place and in the morning it has a fermented, slightly bubbly texture. This mixture can then be used to make porridge or pancakes.

Souring

Sourdough wheat and rye breads contain minimal phytates because these grains have high levels of phytase which is activated by souring. Sourdough bread does still contain gluten, however.

Salad dressings

Dressings make salads more appealing, they bind them together flavour-wise, and they add good fats to make the salads more filling and better for blood sugar. The right kinds of dressings, including home-made mayonnaise, can definitely be considered a health food, and they shouldn't make you put on weight – quite the reverse – as they are good for the metabolism.

Olive oil and apple cider vinegar dressing

This dressing gives you a double-dose of health benefits, since it contains both heart-friendly olive oil and apple cider vinegar. Apple cider vinegar is anti-bacterial, it contains bone and muscle-friendly calcium and magnesium, it strengthens immunity, it aids digestion of protein, it is alkalising, it relieves sore throats and sinus infections, it is a natural appetite suppressant, and it can erase the symptoms of arthritis. It also makes a delicious dressing which goes well with most salads; I also pour it on steamed vegetables to give them a bit of zing.

Ingredients:

3 tablespoons extra-virgin olive oil
1 tablespoon apple cider vinegar
1 teaspoon dijon mustard
1 small garlic clove, chopped small or minced (optional)
Salt and pepper to taste

Method:

Shake the ingredients together in a jar or salad dressing bottle with a tight lid until well blended.

Olive oil and lemon dressing

This goes well with any salad served with meat or fish, and the lemon juice will help you to digest the meat by breaking down the protein. For salads accompanying fish or shellfish, you can also add a squeeze of lime.

Ingredients:

6 tablespoons extra-virgin olive oil (or 3 parts oil to one part lemon juice)
2 tablespoons lemon juice
½-1 clove garlic, chopped small or minced (optional)
Salt and pepper to taste
½ teaspoon honey (optional)

Method:

Shake the ingredients together until well-blended.

Balsamic sesame dressing

Ingredients:

6 tablespoons extra-virgin olive oil (or 3 parts oil to one part vinegar)
2 tablespoons balsamic vinegar
½-1 teaspoon mustard (dijon or coarse grain)
½ clove garlic, chopped small or minced
2-3 teaspoons sesame seeds
½ teaspoon honey (optional)
Salt and pepper to taste

Method:

Dry-fry the sesame seeds in a frying pan for approximately one minute on a medium heat. Meanwhile, shake together the rest of the ingredients in a jar. Add the hot sesame seeds and mix in – they will crackle satisfyingly and imbue the dressing with their flavour.

Mayonnaise

Home-made mayonnaise has health-giving ingredients and it tastes sublime – totally different from processed mayonnaise. All that whisking is good exercise too.

There are many mayonnaise recipes out there and this is just one – my only stipulations are that you should try to use an organic egg, and either olive oil or a mix of olive oil and cold-pressed unrefined sunflower oil.

If you want to make *aioli*, use the same method and ingredients but this time the garlic must be included and it is best to use extra-virgin olive oil or a mix of olive oil and extra-virgin olive oil.

Ingredients:

1 free-range, organic egg yolk at room temperature
1 tablespoon freshly-squeezed lemon juice, apple cider vinegar, or white wine vinegar
1 teaspoon Dijon mustard
1 cup olive oil or ½ cup olive oil mixed with ½ cup unrefined, cold-pressed sunflower oil, in a jug with a spout
A pinch of salt
½ clove garlic (optional)

Method:

Crush the garlic into a paste (if you are using it) and mix with the salt. Mix together the egg yolk, mustard, and vinegar or lemon in a bowl and mix in the garlic and salt. Add a few drops of the oil to the egg yolk, whisking all the time (you will need a good whisk, unless you have a food processor which can do the job). When it is mixed in, add a few more drops, and so on. At some point the mixture should start to have the texture of mayonnaise, at which point you can start adding the oil slightly more quickly. If it splits, add a tablespoon of boiling water to re-emulsify it, and if it becomes too thin, add a tablespoon of warm water to thin it. If you need more oil, add it. By the end you should have a glossy, creamy mayonnaise.

Japanese dressing

Ingredients:

2 tablespoons sesame seeds
2 tablespoons tamari soya sauce
2 tablespoons rice vinegar
1-2 tablespoons cold-pressed ground nut oil
A squeeze of lemon or lime

Method:

Dry-fry the sesame seeds in a pan for around one minute, then mix with the other ingredients.

Salads

Salads are a great staple because they are quick to make, they are an excellent source of nutrients, and they are very versatile – just throw in whatever raw vegetables you have, and then add some proteins, good fats, and maybe a carb. They are perfect for taking to the office – just make a dressing and keep it in a jar, and don't forget the fork as I always do.

Avocado sesame salad

Avocados are a perfect match with chicken, so this goes very well with cold chicken added to the salad or as an accompaniment to a hot chicken dish.

Ingredients (serves 1–2):

1 avocado, sliced
1 carrot, sliced
1/2 cup fine green beans
1 cup salad leaves
1/2 cup rocket
Balsamic sesame dressing, as above

Method:

Toss the salad ingredients together and mix with the dressing just before serving.

Greek salad

This is a staple in the Longevity Hot Spot, the beautiful Greek island of Symi, where capers are revered for their digestive benefits; the herbs add interest and have antiviral and antioxidant power. This salad goes well with fresh sardines to make a meal of its own, and it is also good served with lamb, chicken or bean dishes.

Ingredients (serves 1–2):

2 fresh tomatoes, sliced
1/2 cucumber, sliced
1/2 onion, sliced thin
1/2 cup black olives
1 tablespoon chopped fresh parsley
1 teaspoon oregano
2 teaspoons capers
1/4 cup feta cheese
Freshly-ground black pepper

Method:

Toss all the ingredients except for the feta cheese with olive oil and vinegar or lemon dressing, and crumble the feta over the top.

Mediterranean salad

This goes well with any meat, chicken, fish or bean dish. You can also add some beans (preferably soaked and cooked, but tinned as an emergency) to make this a filling lunch for the office or at home.

Ingredients (serves 2):

½ cup green beans, lightly steamed
½ cup broccoli, cut into florets (raw or very lightly steamed)
A handful of lettuce leaves – whatever good-quality, local, seasonal lettuce you can obtain
A handful of rocket leaves or basil, torn into pieces
A handful of black olives, pitted
3-4 artichoke hearts, from a jar or marinated
1 tablespoon sundried tomatoes, chopped (optional)
1 tablespoon feta cheese, crumbled (optional)

Method:

Mix together the salad ingredients with a dressing of your choice.

Roasted red pepper salad

These are wonderful as a side dish or mixed with a green salad. You can do a large batch of them and keep them covered with olive oil in the refrigerator.

Ingredients (serves 1- 2):

2 red peppers

Juice of one lemon, freshly-squeezed
1/2 -1 clove garlic (optional)
Extra-virgin olive oil
A few pieces of basil, torn

Method:

Either put the peppers under the grill or roast them on a baking tray in a fairly hot oven (160-180C). When the skin is starting to blister and they are getting brown on one side, turn them until they are the same all over. When they are done, put them in a plastic bag and tie the bag. When they are cool, remove the skins (they should come off easily) and open them up and remove the seeds, but try to keep the juices which have a lot of flavour. Tear the peppers into strips and mix with the other ingredients.

Avocado prawns

This isn't exactly a salad, more a variation on the classic Seventies starter, but as it is such a nutrient-rich, easy, tasty dish which could count as a salad I am putting it in here.

Ingredients (serves 1-2):

1 avocado, cut in half and with the stone removed
1 cup prawns, preferably organic, cooked and shelled
Olive oil and apple cider vinegar salad dressing or home-made mayonnaise
½-1 clove garlic, minced or chopped small
The juice of one lime
1 tablespoon coriander, chopped

Method:

Put the prawns in a dish and stir in the garlic and lime juice. Leave for 20 minutes. Place each avocado half on a plate and pour some salad dressing into the well in the centre of the avocado. Put the prawns over the top and sprinkle with the coriander.

Beetroot and carrot salad

This is a colourful salad, and where you have colour, you have nutrients, combining in a synergistic way. Putting this on a table with a green salad looks beautiful and gets the digestive juices going.

Ingredients (serves 2):

1-2 beetroot, uncooked, peeled, and julienned or shredded
2 large carrots, washed or peeled and julienned or grated
2 tablespoons coriander, chopped small
2-3 tablespoons mix of pumpkin and sunflower seeds

Method:

Roast the seeds in the oven at 140 C for ten minutes or dry-fry them in a pan for a minute. Mix with the rest of the ingredients and apple cider vinegar dressing.

Japanese salad

The long-lived Okinawans love their radishes and colourful, beautifully-arranged salads. This recipe goes well with Japanese dishes as well as with the Okinawan staple, the sweet potato. For a quick lunch or office salad, add pieces of cold chicken, aduki beans, quinoa, or mung beans for extra protein.

Ingredients (serves 2-3):

2 spring onions, chopped
5-6 radishes, julienned, sliced, or cut into ribbons
¼ cucumber, with seeds removed, julienned or cut into ribbons
½ cup mange-touts, raw or lightly steamed
1-2 carrots, julienned or cut into ribbons
1 stick celery, chopped small

1 cup sprouts (any kind, eg mung bean sprouts, alfalfa sprouts, broccoli sprouts)

Method:

Mix together the ingredients – if you have a spiraliser you can use this to make ribbons with the radishes, cucumber and carrots – and serve with Japanese dressing (as above).

Crudités and Dips

Dips are a great way to boost your intake of vegetables in a way that is purely pleasurable. If you use raw vegetable crudités as dippers you'll boost your intake even more. If you like having a pre-dinner drink, this is the perfect time for crudités and dips. Try cutting pieces of carrot, celery, cucumber, cauliflower, red pepper, broccoli or any other raw vegetables and serving them with one of these dips.

Guacamole

Guacamole is a favourite in South America, including the Longevity Hot Spot Nicoya in Costa Rica, and it is rich in good fats, vitamin E, and antioxidants. Guacamole is the perfect addition to salads, bean dishes, tortillas, pitta bread, or as a dip with raw carrots.

Ingredients:

1-2 large avocados, mashed with a fork
1-2 tablespoons coriander, finely chopped
1 tomato, finely chopped
1 small onion, finely chopped
The juice of one lime (use a lemon if you have no limes)
1 small chilli pepper, finely chopped (optional)
A pinch of salt

Method:

You can either mix the ingredients together as they are, or you can first pound the onion, coriander, chilli pepper, tomato and salt in a pestle and mortar before mixing with the avocado and lime juice. The guacamole should be a little bit lumpy.

Salsa

This is another Costa Rican favourite. Having salsa as an accompaniment to your dishes will add not only an exciting bit of flavour but also some powerful health benefits. The tomatoes provide the antioxidant lycopene, the onions and garlic are immune-boosting, the chilli peppers contain anti-inflammatory, anti-bacterial capsaicin, the lime provides vitamin C, and the coriander is very high in antioxidants. Salsa is also low in calories, but will boost the feeling of satiety due to its high nutrient content.

Ingredients:

1-2 cloves garlic, peeled and finely chopped or minced
1 onion, finely chopped
3 large ripe tomatoes, chopped small
1-2 chilli peppers, chopped small
3 tablespoons coriander, finely chopped
The juice of one lime
Pepper and a little salt, to taste

Method:

Combine the ingredients in a bowl. If the mixture seems too dry you can add a splash of water. Refrigerate for 2-4 hours to combine the flavours. Serve with Mexican dishes, tapas, as a dip, with guacamole, or any way you like.

Tsatziki

Tsatziki, ubiquitous in Greece, can be used as a dip, as a salad dressing or as a side-dish and goes particularly well with lamb. The Greeks, including the long-lived people of Symi, usually use strained goat's or sheep's milk yoghurt.

Ingredients:

1 cucumber, peeled and with seeds removed, finely chopped or grated
1/2 tablespoon extra virgin olive oil
1 cup plain live yoghurt
Lemon juice
Crushed garlic
Dill or mint
Salt

Method:

Place the cucumber in a sieve with a sprinkle of salt and let it yield some of its juice. This changes the taste of the cucumber and gives tsatziki its essential flavour, so do not miss this stage out. You may also wish to strain the yoghurt so that the tsatsiki is not too liquid; alternatively you can use Greek yoghurt. Pat the cucumber dry with a clean towel then mix with the olive oil and yoghurt. Add lemon juice, garlic, dill ormint according to taste, and a small pinch of salt if required.

Hummus

Hummus is a very versatile dip which can also be used as a sandwich filling, an accompaniment to salads, or a side dish. Hummus provides beneficial fats and protein – if you have sprouted chick peas you will absorb the protein better (see Proteins Week). It is best to make your own, which is incredibly quick and easy, as you then know that it will not contain any dodgy oils – just pure olive oil.

Ingredients:

400g chick peas, preferably soaked and cooked or sprouted –
otherwise use a tin
2-3 heaped tablespoons tahini
The juice of 1-2 lemons (to taste)
½-1 cup olive oil
1-2 cloves garlic, minced
Sea salt

Method:

Blend all the ingredients together to the required taste and
consistency.

Vegetables

Vegetables do not have to be bland and boring. Here are some
suggestions for preparing vegetables in ways to keep them
good-tasting and nutritious.

Oven-roasted vegetables

Roughly chop vegetables suitable for roasting such as squash,
pumpkin, sweet potato, parsnips, beetroot, potato, leeks, fennel,
carrots, onion, and/or garlic. Place them in a baking dish with
a tablespoon of water and a drizzle of peanut oil or a knob of
ghee or butter. Roast on a low heat, stirring occasionally, until
done. Towards the end of roasting you can also add herbs such
as rosemary or thyme.

Stir-fried vegetables

Slice vegetables suitable for stir-frying such as carrot, pak choi,
mange-touts, green beans, peppers, broccoli, cauliflower, onion
and garlic. Stir-fry in groundnut oil and tamari soy sauce or
coconut oil, or 'healthy sauté' (see Fats Week for instructions)
in a small amount of stock, using a frying pan or wok. Cook

for a short time – just a few minutes at the most - so that the vegetables still have crunch and bite.

Steamed vegetables

Steaming vegetables for a short time is better than boiling since minerals are not lost into the water. It is also very quick and easy. Green vegetables, carrots, and sweet potatoes all lend themselves well to steaming. Just a few minutes is enough – keep the vegetables crunchy and green. Serve with a drizzle of olive oil and/or a knob of butter, garlic, lemon, and seasoning, or with apple cider vinegar dressing. You can also grate a little parmesan over steamed vegetables such as broccoli, mange-touts, green beans and asparagus.

Fermented vegetables

If you feel adventurous, you may like to have a go at making your own fermented vegetables. You may, of course, be an old hand already. I have to confess I have never tried making my own sauerkraut, because the health food shop near me sells four different varieties. The internet has many websites devoted to the subject, so I suggest consulting one of those. All you need is a cabbage and/or other vegetables, salt, and a jar.

Soups

Soups are very versatile and easy to improvise, and they make a good receptacle for ingredients you have hanging around the kitchen not getting used. If you don't have one, it is worth investing in a soup thermos so that you can take soup into work or outside in cold weather.

Leftover vegetable soup

This is an excellent way to use up vegetables being neglected at the bottom of the refrigerator – the soup can then be frozen and used as and when it is needed. If you have chicken stock from leftover roast chicken, that's even better. I recently discovered that in Vietnamese cooking, stock is left to simmer for around 17 hours, so I started making chicken stock from leftover roast chicken in the slow cooker, leaving it overnight or longer, and it tastes amazing.

Ingredients (serves 1-2):

2-3 cups of any leftover vegetables you have (eg broccoli, spinach, carrots, potatoes, sweet potatoes, leeks, cauliflower, parsnips etc)
1 onion, chopped small
1-2 cloves garlic
3-4 cups chicken or vegetable stock (from real stock or organic cubes)
1-2 teaspoons mixed dried herbs
A knob of butter or ghee (optional)
Extra-virgin olive oil
Live plain yoghurt (optional)

Method:

Cook the onion in a heavy-based pan using the 'healthy sauté method', adding the butter or ghee if you want to. Stir for a few minutes until the vegetables are softening, then add the herbs and stir in. Cover with stock, bring to the boil, and simmer until the vegetables are soft. Blend to the desired consistency and serve drizzled with olive oil and a dollop of live plain yoghurt.

Roasted root vegetable soup

This is a great way to use up leftover roasted vegetables. Celeriac, parsnips, sweet potatoes, onion and carrot all work perfectly – just follow the instructions as above, but using roasted root vegetables instead of fresh ones. The cooking time will of course be shorter. If you have leftover roast chicken you can add that too, and use real chicken stock from the carcass.

Thai sweet potato and carrot soup

This soup is high in beta-carotene from the orange vegetables, and so is good for the immune system, especially of the respiratory and gastro-intestinal tracts as beta-carotene is converted to vitamin A which protects these areas.

Ingredients (serves 2):

2 sweet potatoes, chopped
2-3 carrots, chopped
1 tablespoon groundnut oil OR ½-1 tablespoon coconut oil OR 2 tablespoons chicken or vegetable stock
1 tin coconut milk
½-1 organic chicken stock cube (optional)
1 tablespoon red Thai curry paste
1 small knob ginger, finely chopped/minced
1 fat clove garlic, finely chopped/minced
The zest and juice of a lime
2 tablespoons coriander, finely chopped
Live plain yoghurt

Method:

Cook the sweet potatoes and carrots in a heavy-based pan. You can use the 'healthy sauté' method for this, or you can use groundnut oil with a splash of water, or you can use coconut oil, depending on your taste preference or what you have available. If you use the 'healthy sauté' method you can use either stock or just plain water.

Cook on a low heat for 5-7 minutes or until the vegetables are starting to soften, stirring from time to time. Add the Thai curry paste, ginger, garlic and lime zest and stir in. Cover the vegetables with water or chicken stock, bring to the boil, and simmer until they are soft. Blend until smooth. Serve with some lime juice, a dollop of live yoghurt, and a sprinkle of coriander.

Coconut mung bean soup

Mung beans are a good bean for bean-lovers to use, because they are lower in anti-nutrients than other beans, especially after soaking, as well as being a good source of protein and fibre.

Ingredients (serves 1-2):

1 onion, grated
1 clove garlic, chopped small or minced
1 stick celery, chopped very small
1 large carrot, grated
1-2 cups mung beans, soaked overnight and cooked
1 cup French beans, chopped
½ cup chicken or vegetable stock
1 tin coconut milk
1-2 teaspoons coconut oil
1 stick lemon grass
1 kaffir lime leaf
1-2 tablespoons coriander stalks
1 teaspoon ginger powder or fresh chopped ginger
The juice of one lime
The juice of one lemon
2 tablespoons coriander, chopped

Method:

Cook the onion in a heavy-based pan either in the coconut oil or using the 'healthy sauté' method. After a couple of minutes, add the garlic, celery, and carrot. Cook for a few minutes, then add the stock, coconut milk, kaffir lime leaf, ginger, coriander stalks and stick of lemon grass. Bring to the boil and simmer for 10-15 minutes. Add the mung beans, green beans, lemon juice and lime juice and simmer for another 5 minutes or until the French beans are cooked. Serve with the chopped coriander sprinkled on top.

Pork, pasta and bean soup

This dish from the Longevity Hot Spot, Campodimele in Italy, has an authentic flavour and should leave you feeling a great sense of satisfaction and well-being, as well as a desire to have it many more times. This goes well with a salad to increase your vegetable intake, and you can leave out the pasta if you prefer.

Ingredients (serves 4):

Approx 200-250g diced organic pork (use the best-quality you can find)
1 carton (around 390g) chopped organic tomatoes OR 4 fresh chopped tomatoes plus 1 tablespoon tomato paste
3 fat cloves garlic, chopped small
1 large onion, chopped finely
1 organic vegetable stock cube or 1/2 tablespoon vegetable stock powder
½ stick celery, chopped small
100g pasta (you can also use brown rice pasta or corn pasta)
75g beans, ideally soaked overnight and cooked rather than tinned (cannelloni beans, fava beans or borlotti beans work well)
75g green beans, sliced

2 teaspoons butter or pork lard (optional)
1 teaspoon mixed Mediterranean herbs
Parmesan, feta, or hard goat's or sheep's cheese
Freshly-ground pepper
Extra-virgin olive oil

Method:

Cook the onion and celery in a heavy-based pan for 2-3 minutes using the 'healthy sauté' method, adding the butter or pork lard if you like. Add the garlic and stir for a minute. Add the stock powder or cube and a tablespoonful of water and stir to dissolve the stock. Add the meat and cook for about 5-10 minutes, or until the meat browns slightly, stirring from time to time. Add the tomatoes, herbs and seasoning and simmer for 4-5 minutes, then add approximately three quarters of a litre of water.

Put the lid on the pan and simmer for 45 minutes. Add the pasta, replace the lid, and simmer until the pasta is 5 minutes from being cooked. Add the green beans and the cooked or tinned beans and simmer for a further 5 minutes. Serve with the grated cheese, a drizzle of olive oil, and a grind of pepper and enjoy with a glass of wine.

Fish soup

This succulent soup from the Longevity Hot Spot, Symi, in Greece has a very attractive rust colour and a beautiful flavour. It goes perfectly with Greek salad and makes a meal of its own.

Ingredients (serves 2-3):

For the fish stock:

Fish for boiling, including the heads and bones (ask your fishmonger what they recommend)

1.2 litres (2 pints) water
1 onion, cut in half
2 sticks celery
1-2 carrots
2 bay leaves
6 peppercorns
A few stalks of flat-leaved parsley
1 teaspoon sea salt

<u>For the soup:</u>

500 g fish suitable for boiling and eating, filleted and cut into fairly large chunks
2 glasses white wine
2 tablespoons olive oil
1 onion, chopped
2-3 cloves garlic, chopped
3 sticks fennel, chopped small
2 large tomatoes, chopped small
1 tablespoon tomato paste
1-2 large potatoes, peeled and sliced into thick slices
The juice of 2 lemons
1 large pinch of saffron
Sea salt and freshly-ground black pepper
A few sprigs of parsley

Method:

To make the fish stock, put all of the ingredients for the stock in a large pan of water, bring to the boil and simmer for about an hour until the juice is reduced by half. Strain, throw out the solids, and keep the stock.

To make the soup, cook the onion, garlic and fennel in a heavy-based pan for 2 minutes using the 'healthy sauté' method – you can use a tablespoonful or two of the fish stock for this. Add a splash more of the fish stock if necessary, put on the lid, and turn the heat right down to let the vegetables sweat for

5 minutes. Add half the fish and stir it in. Add the wine, turn up the heat, and cook until the wine has reduced by half. Add the tomatoes, tomato paste and lemon juice, and cook for 3-4 minutes. Cover with the fish stock and simmer until the liquid has reduced by half. Add the saffron, season to taste, and add more lemon juice if required. Put in the sliced potatoes and the rest of the fish, and cook for 10-15 minutes or until the potatoes are ready. Remove from the heat, stir in the olive oil, and serve garnished with parsley.

Pork noodles with dashi

For the dashi

Dashi is a sauce used as the basis for many Japanese and Okinawan dishes. It is very easy to make, but tastes authentically subtle-yet-complex; delicate-yet-satisfying.

Ingredients:

2 strips kombu seaweed
Approx. 5g bonito flakes (available in sachets from oriental food retailers)
1 tablespoon tamari soya sauce or good-quality soya sauce

Method:

Boil the kombu for 3-4 minutes in about half a pint of water. Remove from the heat. Add the bonito flakes and return to the heat. Remove the pan from the heat again just as the water comes to the boil. Leave to stand for 5 minutes or until the bonito flakes sink. Strain and reserve the liquid. Discard the solids (they can be reused if you are making a second batch of dashi the same day). Add the soy sauce.

<u>For the soup:</u>

Ingredients (serves 1–2):

Approx 100-150g pork, sliced in thin strips
½ clove garlic
1 tablespoon dashi
1-2 teaspoons tamari or soy sauce
¾ teaspoon sake, mirin or sweet white wine
I cup pork stock (you will make this first with the pork)
100g Asian noodles such as buckwheat or udon noodles
3 stalks spring onions (scallions), chopped very fine

Method:

Boil the pork in about half a litre of water for 25 minutes. Skim the fat off the top of the stock and put it aside – you can use it for the next step. The rest of the stock goes in the soup.

Whilst boiling the pork, cook the noodles in a separate pan, strain, and set aside. Alternatively, if the noodles are quick to cook, you can cook them in the soup at the end.

Heat half a tablespoonful of the pork fat in a wok or frying pan. Add the garlic and sauté gently, without letting it brown.

Add the pork and stir for a few seconds. Add the dashi, soy, sake and stock and bring to the boil. Add the noodles and heat through (if pre-cooked) or cook. Garnish with the onion and serve.

Miso soup with tofu, chicken and noodles

This is a warming, quick soup with two protein sources in it as well as vegetables so it makes a meal in itself. Adding the miso after turning off the heat means that the probiotics in the miso are more likely to survive. If you are carb-free, you can leave out the noodles.

Ingredients (serves 2):

100g noodles (*e.g.* buckwheat, udon, or brown rice)
50g tofu, cut into cubes
50-100g chicken, cut into small pieces
1 small onion or shallot, chopped very small
1 clove garlic, chopped
1 teaspoon ground or chopped ginger (optional)
2-3 cups water or chicken stock
1/2 cup broccoli, chopped
1/2 cup green beans, sliced
1 tablespoon soya sauce (preferably tamari soya sauce or other good-quality type)
1 heaped tablespoon miso paste
2 teaspoons sesame oil
1 tablespoon chopped coriander

Method:

Cook the noodles as directed, leaving them slightly under-cooked so that they do not become over-cooked in the hot soup. Drain and put to one side, rinsing them if they are starchy. Cook the onion or shallot for 1-2 minutes using the 'healthy sauté' method. Add the tofu, chicken, garlic and ginger if you are using it and cook for about 30 seconds. Add the water or stock and bring to the boil. Add the vegetables and cook for 3-4 minutes until the vegetables are just cooked. Take off the heat and stir in the sesame oil, tamari and miso paste. Add the noodles and serve with the chopped coriander sprinkled on top. Add additional tamari sauce to taste if necessary.

Main dishes

Oven-roasted salmon

Ingredients (serves 2):
2 pieces of the best-quality salmon you can find, preferably

from a fishmonger (try Norwegian Var salmon if you can get
it; some Irish organic salmon is also excellent)
Butter
A pinch of sea salt (optional)
Half a lemon, cut into slices
2 lemon wedges
1 tablespoon dill, chopped (optional)
Mayonnaise (preferably home-made)

Method:

Pre-heat the oven to 190 C. Put a piece of tinfoil in an oven
dish and place the salmon pieces on top. Put a knob of butter
on them and a pinch of salt if you like, the dill if you are using
it, and lay a few slices of lemon on top. Wrap the foil loosely
over the fish. Cook for approximately 30 minutes, checking
to make sure that the fish isn't overcooked – it should stay
succulent and moist (if the pieces of salmon are small the
cooking time may be shorter, or longer if they are large). Serve
with the mayonnaise and lemon wedges, plus a good heap of
vegetables.

Baked fish in wine

This is a popular way of cooking fish in the Longevity Hot
Spot, Symi in Greece. Since it involves heating olive oil, it
is best to use ordinary olive oil rather than extra-virgin olive
oil; oil expert George Mateljan states that ordinary olive oil
is used for cooking in the Mediterranean as it contains fewer
polyphenols which become damaged by heat than extra-virgin
olive oil.

This dish goes very well with a Greek salad or green salad
and if you want to have it with carbs, potatoes, rice or quinoa
are good options. In Symi it is often accompanied by home-
made bread dipped in olive oil.

Ingredients (serves 2-3):

Requires 1 hour refrigeration time before cooking
1 large fresh fish suitable for baking (monkfish, bass or any white fish works well)
2-3 tablespoons fresh parsley, chopped
1-2 large cloves garlic, chopped small
1 lemon
5 or 6 ripe, red tomatoes
2 onions, sliced
1 green pepper, cut into strips
1 yellow pepper, cut into strips
1 red pepper, cut into strips
240 ml (8 fl oz) olive oil
1 large glass of white wine
Sea salt and freshly-ground black pepper

Method:

Clean and wash the fish if necessary. Season both sides of the fish, stuff the belly with the parsley and garlic, then squeeze the lemon over the fish. Refrigerate for one hour.

Put half the tomatoes, onions and peppers in a baking dish in a layer, place the fish on top, then put a second layer of the vegetables on top. Pour over the olive oil. Bake at 200 C for 15 minutes. Baste the mixture with the juices. Add the wine, and bake for another 15 minutes.

Fish bites in gluten-free breadcrumbs

I have included this because it is always a dead cert with children, and is superior both in taste and nutrient content to frozen fishfingers.

Ingredients (serves 2):

200-300g filleted, skinless white fish, such as cod or haddock

75g gluten-free breadcrumbs (available from health food shops)
1 organic, free range egg
3-4 tablespoons groundnut oil
1 lemon
A pinch of salt

Method:

Cut the fish into bite-sized pieces. You can marinade it for 20-30 minutes in the juice of the lemon at this point if you wish. Beat the egg in a bowl and put the breadcrumbs on a plate, mixing them with the salt if you wish. Dip each fish piece into the egg, then roll it in the breadcrumbs. Heat the oil in a frying pan and add the fish pieces. Cook for 2-3 minutes each side or until done. Serve with lemon wedges (or, worst case scenario, tomato ketchup) and lots of vegetables.

Chicken in miso and tamari

This is an easy way to make chicken taste a bit more interesting and it goes well with a good heap of vegetables. Try steamed or stir-fried broccoli, carrots, sugar-snap pea, French beans, and/or cauliflower. If you want to have it with carbs, brown rice noodles with tamari soya sauce and garlic work well.

Ingredients (serves 2):

2 chicken breasts or 2-4 chicken thighs and drumsticks, preferably from an organic, free-range chicken
1-2 tablespoons miso paste
2 tablespoons tamari soya sauce
1 lemon (optional)

Method:

Put the chicken in an oven dish and spread with the miso, then add the tamari. Cook at 180 C for around 45 minutes or until done. Serve with lemon wedges.

Slow-cooked casserole

I recently bought a slow cooker, which I use sometimes in winter. Slow-cooking isn't actually the ideal way to cook in terms of vitamin content, but the minerals at least are retained. The best thing about it is that you have to do minimal preparation and you can go out for the day and come back to find a lovely casserole waiting for you. The flavour is also much better for the long cooking time. And if you make sure to add vegetables at the end and serve it with a big salad, you will get a good nutrient intake that way.

This goes well with baked potatoes, sweet potatoes, brown rice or quinoa. It is best to use chopped tomatoes from a carton or jar, or fresh ones, rather than from a tin as tinned tomatoes can be high in harmful chemicals.

Ingredients (serves 3-4):

Approx 300g chicken or lamb, preferably organic and free-range
400g beans, (eg black beans, kidney beans, cannelloni beans) preferably soaked overnight and dried but otherwise tinned (these can be as well as or instead of the meat, or you can leave them out)
2 cartons (approx. 390g each) chopped tomatoes with juice
1 onion, chopped
1 stick celery, chopped
2-3 cloves garlic, chopped small
1-2 carrots, chopped small
1 red pepper, chopped small
½ tablespoon vegetable bouillon or a stock cube dissolved in water
2 teaspoons mixed dried herbs
100g frozen petits pois
100g French beans
2 tablespoons extra-virgin olive oil

Method:

Put everything apart from the beans (if you are using them), peas and French beans in the slow cooker. If you want to, you can brown the meat first in a frying pan in a knob of butter or ghee or a little groundnut oil – this will add flavour to the casserole. If you do this, get the rest of the ingredients hot first by putting them in the slow cooker on the 'high' setting for 20 minutes or so before you add the browned meat.

Cook for around 4 hours if using the 'high' setting or 6-7 hours if using the 'low' setting. Cooking times can be approximate, and you don't have to stir the casserole but you can give it the occasional stir if you happen to be nearby. About 30 minutes before serving, add the beans and green vegetables. Mix the olive oil in at the end.

Liver and onions

Some people like liver, some people don't. Some people think they don't like it but are willing to give it another try when they discover a) how nutrient-rich it is and b) how cheap it is – try to find a good butcher who can supply you with top-quality organic stuff. Liver is an excellent source of vitamins and minerals, including vitamin A which protects gut and respiratory tract health. Avoid non-organic liver, since it can be high in toxins.

Serve your liver with a few helpings of vegetables and a carb if you wish. I find that carrots and spinach go particularly well with liver – you get extra vitamin A that way too.

Ingredients (serves 2):

3-4 strips of organic lamb or calf liver
1 onion, sliced fairly thin
1 knob ghee or butter/1-2 teaspoons groundnut oil (optional)

Method:

Cook the onions in a frying pan using the 'healthy sauté' method. When they are getting soft, add the liver – if there isn't enough juice in the pan from the onions you can add the ghee, butter or groundnut oil at this stage to stop the liver from sticking. Cook for around 5 minutes on each side, and season to taste.

Lamb, pasta and feta stew

A version of this, known as *daudo*, is eaten on special occasions in the Longevity Hot Spot, Hunza in Pakistan, only using strips of chapatti rather than pasta, and their own similar version of feta cheese. There are lots of good things in here, and the fat is removed from the meat juices, as is the custom in most of the Longevity Hot Spots.

If you don't want to make this with pasta, use quinoa, brown rice, or barley instead, served on the side.

Ingredients (serves 2):

200g chunks of lamb
2 onions, one whole and one chopped very small or shredded
3 cloves garlic, chopped
1 stick celery, chopped very small
6-8 tomatoes, chopped very small
2 tablespoons tomato purée
100g pasta (tagliatelle broken into shorter pieces works well)
2 teaspoons oregano or mixed herbs
Sea salt and freshly ground pepper to taste
50g organic feta cheese
1 tablespoon extra-virgin olive oil
A glass of wine (optional)

Method:

Boil the lamb in a pan of water with the onion for about an hour to create stock.

When the stock is almost ready, cook the onion, garlic and celery in a heavy-based pan using the 'healthy sauté' method until they are soft. Remove the meat from the stock, add it to the vegetables, and cook for a few minutes. Add the tomatoes with the tomato purée and cook for another 5-10 minutes.

Skim the fat from the top of the stock and add enough to the vegetables so that the liquid level is about an inch above the solids. Simmer with the lid on for about an hour. Add more juice if necessary. You can also add a glass of red or white wine. Add the pasta and cook until it is *al dente*. Add the herbs and season with a pinch of salt and pepper to taste. Mix in the olive oil and serve with the feta cheese crumbled over the top.

Black bean gluten-free lasagne

I adapted this from a vegetarian lasagne recipe somebody gave me. It does involve dairy, but the combination of cheeses with the brown rice lasagne sheets is delicious, and at least there's no gluten or white sauce. This always goes perfectly with a big green salad.

Ingredients (serves 2):

400g black beans, preferably soaked overnight and cooked (but, if necessary, from a tin)
1 large onion, chopped small
1 stick celery, chopped small
1 red pepper, chopped small
1 courgette, chopped small
1 carrot, chopped small
½ tablespoon vegetable stock powder or 1 vegetable stock cube
1 carton chopped tomatoes (around 390g)
2 tablespoons tomato paste

1-2 teaspoons dried mixed herbs

Approx 150-200g organic cottage cheese

Approx 50g organic hard cheese (eg sheep's cheese or cheddar cheese)

Approx 8 sheets brown rice lasagne (if you can't get it you can try to find another gluten-free variety or use ordinary lasagne if you wish)

Method:

Cook the vegetables in a heavy-based pan using the 'healthy sauté' method, with the stock powder or cube mixed into a couple of tablespoonsful of water. When they are soft, add the chopped tomatoes, tomato paste and herbs and simmer for 10 minutes with the lid on to keep the moisture in. Add the beans and simmer for another 5 minutes. You can then leave this mixture overnight if you want to, so as to let the flavours all blend into each other, or you can move straight to the next step.

Soak your brown rice lasagne sheets in hot water for a few minutes or as directed to soften them slightly, or par-boil them for half a minute. Put a layer of the bean mixture in the bottom of the lasagne dish, then cover with a layer of lasagne sheets. Add another layer of bean mixture, and another layer of lasagne. If there is still more bean mixture you can do this one more time. Spread the cottage cheese over the top layer of lasagne and grate the hard cheese over the top. Cover with tinfoil and cook in a preheated oven at 180 C for 30 minutes, then remove the tinfoil and cook for another 5-10 minutes.

Brown rice mushroom risotto

I have included this recipe not to encourage you to eat large amounts of stodge or grains, but because if you are a risotto-lover, I recommend using short-grain brown rice rather than white risotto rice as it gives the risotto a fuller flavour and will

215

be less bad for blood sugar levels. Rather than having it as a main dish, try having it as an adjunct to a large salad and a protein food such as chicken or a bean dish.

Ingredients (serves 2–4):

1 onion, chopped small
1 or 2 cloves garlic, chopped
2 carrots, peeled and chopped
2 celery stalks, chopped
2 cups mushrooms – any type, sliced (porcini mushrooms are best for flavour; if using dried porcini mushrooms, soak in hot water and retain the stock to use for cooking the risotto)
1 cup short grain brown rice
½ tablespoon butter, lard or ghee
8 oz. white or red wine
2 cups organic chicken or vegetable stock
2 tablespoons extra-virgin olive oil
Freshly-ground black pepper
Parmesan cheese, preferably organic
1-2 teaspoons mixed dried herbs

Method:

Boil the rice for 10 minutes to partially cook it – don't miss this part out, or you will find yourself stirring your risotto for a very long time and getting a sore bicep. Cook half of the mushrooms in the butter, lard or ghee for 4-5 minutes and put aside. Cook the onions for 2-3 minutes in a heavy-based pan using the 'healthy sauté' method. Add the garlic and cook for a minute. Add the carrots and celery and continue to cook, stirring constantly, for 4-5 minutes. Add the uncooked mushrooms and cook for a minute. Raise the heat and add the brown rice. Let it crackle for a few seconds. If you are using wine, add it now and mix it into the rice, letting it sizzle.

Add a ladle of the stock and stir it into the rice until it is absorbed. Keep adding the stock one ladle at a time in this way. Keep the heat on medium/low so that the risotto is just simmering. Keep stirring all the time. When the rice is cooked (this will take about 45 minutes so you will need to listen to the radio and drink a glass of wine at the same time) add the rest of the cooked mushrooms and stir through. Add the olive oil, herbs, black pepper, and a modest amount of grated Parmesan cheese.

Corn tortillas with black beans and guacamole

This and *gallo pinto* (rice and beans) form the main staple dishes in the Longevity Hot Spot, Nicoya, in Costa Rica and are frequently eaten three times a day, usually with guacamole and salsa on the side, as well as a type of sour yoghurt. A green leafy salad goes well with this too.

Ideally, make your own tortillas from nixtamalised corn flour (*masa*), if you can get it. I get mine from a Mexican shop in Bristol, where it is shipped over from Mexico. They also have purple masa from a particular variety of corn, which looks beautiful with the other colours on the plate.

If you can't get hold of masa flour, you can use bought tortillas, but they are usually made with white flour and have preservatives added. Alternatively, you can have the beans with quinoa, a baked potato, or brown rice.

Ingredients (serves 2):

4 small tortillas, or 2 large ones
1-2 cups refried beans (see Breakfast Week for the recipe)
Soured cream, preferably organic
Guacamole (as above, under 'Dips')
Salsa (as above, under 'Dips')
2 tablespoons coriander, chopped

Method:

If you can get hold of masa flour, make the dough by mixing the flour with warm water and kneading it into a dough as directed, then leave it, covered, for 15 minutes. If you can also get hold of a tortilla press, it is easy to make perfect tortillas by shaping some dough into a little ball and flattening it in the press. Heat the tortillas in a dry pan for 2-3 minutes each side.

Meanwhile, heat up your refried beans. When the tortillas are ready, place the bean mixture in the centre of the tortilla, add a dollop of guacamole and soured cream, sprinkle with coriander, fold, and eat. Serve with the salsa on the side.

Less-bad toasted cheese sandwich

If you feel the need for a toastie, this at least has more taste and nutrient value than your bland white-bread-and-processed-cheese kind; when I indulge I have it with a big helping of green salad with cider vinegar dressing.

Ingredients:

2 slices whole grain wheat or rye bread (preferably sourdough)
1-2 teaspoons tomato paste
½ clove garlic, minced
½ teaspoon mixed herbs
1-2 slices cheese (preferably organic – I use sheep's cheese)
Olive oil
½ tomato, sliced

Method:

Drizzle a little olive oil on your bread then spread with tomato paste. Spread the crushed garlic into the tomato paste and sprinkle with herbs. Add the cheese and tomato slices. Either cook in a toasted sandwich maker or under the grill. If you use a toasted sandwich-maker, you may need to use a little oil to prevent sticking – the oil will get hot, so try not to use too much. Serve with a large helping of salad.

Dhal with lemon and coriander

Dhal is a staple of the Longevity Hot Spot, Hunza in Pakistan. Lentils are not well-digested by everybody, but if you are someone who finds they agree with you when they are properly-prepared, then this recipe makes a great side-dish. Hunzakuts crumble home-made brown bread into their dhal; an alternative is to eat it with brown rice, quinoa, or sourdough bread on the side.

Ingredients (serves 2):

400g lentils (brown, black or yellow), soaked, rinsed, and cooked
1 large onion, shredded
½ tablespoon ghee or butter (optional)
3 tomatoes, chopped very small
2 tablespoons tomato paste
2-3 fresh green chilli peppers, chopped small
2 teaspoons garam masala or curry powder
½-1 organic chicken stock cube dissolved in a little water
Sea salt (optional)
The juice of 2 lemons
1 bunch coriander, chopped
2-4 tablespoons plain live yoghurt or *raita*

Method:

Cook the onion for 3-4 minutes or until soft in a heavy-based pan using the 'healthy sauté' method; you can use the ghee or butter here if you like. Add the tomatoes, tomato paste, stock and chillis and cook for around 5 minutes, stirring occasionally. Add the garam masala or curry powder and a little salt to taste if desired.

Add the cooked lentils to the mixture and simmer for 5 minutes. Add extra tomato paste and/or water if the dhal is too dry. Squeeze in the lemon juice, then mix in the coriander and serve with the yoghurt or *raita* on the side.

Aduki bean burgers

This is one of those recipes with which you can experiment with endless variations of your own. Try adding sun-dried tomatoes, chilli pepper, mustard, cheese, or different herbs, for example. Serve with a big green salad.

Ingredients (serves 2-3):

2 cups aduki beans, preferably soaked overnight and cooked (otherwise tinned)
1 cup millet or quinoa, cooked
1 red onion, chopped very small
1 stick celery, chopped very small
1 carrot, chopped very small
1-2 cloves garlic, minced
1 tablespoon parsley or coriander, chopped small
2 tablespoons groundnut oil
Sea salt and freshly-ground black pepper

Method:

Cook the red onion and garlic for 2-3 minutes using the 'healthy saute' method, then add the rest of the vegetables and cook for a further 5 minutes until soft. Remove from the heat and put the mixture into a food processor. Add the quinoa, aduki beans and oil and blend until they are well-combined. Add the parsley or coriander, pepper to taste and a pinch of salt if required and whizz round once more to mix in.

Put the mixture in a bowl and refrigerate it for 30-60 minutes. Remove and form into small patties – to do this, make a ball and then flatten it slightly between your palms.

Place the burgers on a lightly-oiled baking tray and cook at 375F/190C/Gas mark 5 for 30 minutes, turning the burgers over once mid-way through cooking.

Snack ideas

During Breakfast Week, you may have found that having a mid-morning or mid-afternoon snack helped keep your blood sugar levels on an even keel. Fruit makes a great snack, but if you need more, have something containing protein and good fats, as this will be very helpful for balancing blood sugar. Here are some ideas:

• Oat cakes or brown rice cakes with hummus
• Oat cakes or brown rice cakes with avocado, carrot and cottage cheese
• Carrots with hummus
• Carrots dipped in nut butter (sugar-free and without hydrogenated vegetable fats)
• Carrots dipped in guacamole
• A handful of nuts and seeds
• A smoothie with added ground flax or chia seeds
• A piece of fruit (try non-sweet fruits such as an apple or orange)

References

How the Stacking Plan can help you

1. Proietto, Joseph et al (2011). Long Term Persistence of Hormonal Adaptations to Weight Loss. *New England Journal of Medicine* 365:1597-1604
2. *ibid.*
3. Hulsegge G, Susan H, Picavet A et al (2013). Today's adult generations are less healthy than their predecessors: Generation shifts in metabolic risk factors: the Doetinchem Cohort Study. *European Journal of Preventive Cardiology*
4. Weingart SN, Ship AN, Aronson MD (2000), Confidential Clinician-reported surveillance of adverse events among medical inpatients; *Journal of General Internal Medicine*, 15 (7): 470-7
5. Starfield Barbara MD, MPH (2000). Is US Health Really the Best in the World? *Journal of the American Medical Association*, July 26, Vol 284 no. 4 p 483
6. Rita F. Redberg, MD; Mitchell H. Katz, MD (2012). Healthy Men Should Not Take Statins
7. *Journal of the American Medical Association* 307(14):1491-1492
8. Tiefer L (2006) Female Sexual Dysfunction: A Case Study of Disease Mongering and Activist Resistance. PLoS Med 3(4): e178. doi:10.1371/journal.pmed.0030178
9. Earl S. Ford, M.D., M.P.H., medical officer, U.S. Public Health Service and U.S. Centers for Disease Control and Prevention, Atlanta; David L. Katz, M.D., director, internal medicine and preventive medicine/public health, Prevention Research Center, Yale University School of Medicine, Derby, Conn.; Aug. 10/24, 2009, *Archives of Internal Medicine*
10. www.webmd.com/cancer/features/top-cancer-fighting-foods

Why and how the Stacking Plan works

1. World Health Organisation, Symposia on Nutrition-Related Chronic Diseases, New Delhi, February 1997. From http://www.searo.who.int/en/Section980/Section1162/Section1167/Section1171_4797.htm
2. Beare, Sally (2005). 50 Secrets of the World's Longest-Living People. (Avalon, USA)
3. *ibid.*
4. Gardner, Jeoffrey P et al (2005). Rise in Insulin Resistance is Associated with Escalated Telomere Attrition. *Circulation*; 111:2171-2177
5. Edwards, T (2005). Inflammation, pain and chronic disease: an integrative approach to treatment and prevention. *Altern Ther Health Med*. 11(6)20-7
6. Whitehead, R., Perrett, D., Ozakinci, G (2012). Appealing to Vanity: Could Potential Appearance Improvement Motivate Fruit and Vegetable Consumption? *American Journal of Public Health*. 102(2):207-211

Breakfast Week

1. Sandercock, G R H; Voss, C and Dye, L (2010). Associations between habitual school-day breakfast consumption, body mass index, physical activity and cardiorespiratory fitness in English schoolchildren *European Journal of Clinical Nutrition* 64, 1086-1092
2. *ibid.*
3. Garaulet M, Gómez-Abellán P (2014). *Physiol Behav*. Timing of food intake and obesity: A novel association
4. Mekary, Rania A et al (2012). Eating patterns and type 2 diabetes risk in men: breakfast omission, eating frequency and snacking. *American Journal of Clinical Nutrition*, March 28
5. Rampersaud GC et al (2005). Breakfast habits, nutritional status, body weight and academic performance in children and adolescents. *Journal of the American Dietetic Association* 105(5): 743-60

Fruit Week

1. Muraki, Isao (2013). Fruit consumption and risk of type 2 diabetes: results from three prospective longitudinal cohort studies. *British Medical Journal* 347:f5001
2. Liu, Rui Hai (2003). Health benefits of fruit and vegetables are from additive and synergistic combinations of phytochemicals. *American Journal of Clinical Nutrition* 78(3);517S-520S
3. Liu, Rui H (2004). Apple phytochemicals and their health benefits. *Nutrition Journal* 3:5
4. *Journal of Agricultural and Food Chemistry,* January 2012.
5. Liu, Rui H (2004). Apple phytochemicals and their health benefits. *Nutrition Journal* 3:5
6. *ibid.*
7. Liu, Rui Hai (2007). Triterpenoids isolated from apple peels have potent anti-proliferative activity and may be partially responsible for apple's anti-cancer activity. *Journal of Agricultural and Food Chemistry* 55(11)4366-4370
8. Schwartz, Steven J (2005). How Can the Metabolomic Response to Lycopene (Exposures, Durations, Intracellular Concentrations) in Humans be Adequately Evaluated? *Journal of Nutrition* 135:2040S-2041S
9. Shukitt-Hale, B; Lau FC; Joseph JA. Berry Fruit Supplementation and the Aging Brain. *Journal of Agricultural and Food Chemistry.* 2008;56:636-641
10. Seymour E Mitchell et al (2011). Blueberry Intake Alters Skeletal Muscle and Adipose Tissue Peroxisome Proliferator-Activated Receptor Activity and Reduces Insulin Resistance in Obese Rats. *Journal of Medicinal Food* 14(12); 1511-1518
11. Tanaka T et al (1993). Inhibition of 4-nitroquinoline-1-oxide induced rat tongue carcinogenesis by the naturally occurring plant phenolics caffeic, ellagic, chlorogenic and ferulic acids. *Carcinogenesis* 14(7):1321-1325
12. Thani NAA, Keshavarz S, Lwaleed BA, et al

(2014). Cytotoxicity of gemcitabine enhanced by polyphenolics from Aronia melanocarpa in pancreatic cancer cell line AsPC-1. *Journal of Clinical Pathology*. Published online September 17 2014

13. Kang (2003), *Journal of Biomedicine and Biotechnology*

14. Zhang Y, et al (2012). Cherry consumption and decreased risk of recurrent gout attacks. *Arthritis Rheum*

15. Fujioka K et al (2006). The effects of grapefruit on weight and insulin resistance: relationship to the metabolic syndrome. *J Med Food* 9(1):49-54

16. Beneficial effects of virgin coconut oil on lipid parameters and in vitro LDL oxidation. *Clin Biochem*. 2004. Sep; 37(9):830-5

17. Anti-tumor effect of medium-chain triglyceride and its influence on the self-defence system of the body. *Cancer Detection and Prevention*. 1998 22(3):219-24

18. Medium-chain fatty acids ameliorate insulin resistance caused by high-fat diets in rats. *Diabetes Metab Res Rev* 2009 Feb 25(2)185-94

19. Mares-Perlman JA, Millen AE, Ficek TL, Hankinson SE (2002). The body of evidence to support a protective role for lutein and zeaxanthin in delaying chronic disease. Overview. *J. Nutr*. 132(3):518S-524S

20. Athar, M et al, (2007). Resveratrol: a review of preclinical human studies for human cancer prevention. *Journal of Applied Toxicology and Clinical Pharmacology* 224(3) 274-283)

21. Forastiere, F et al (2000). Consumption of fresh fruit rich in vitamin C and wheezing symptoms in children. *Thorax* 55:283-288

22. Saleem, M et al (2004). Lupeol modulates NF Kappa B and P13K/Akt pathways and inhibits skin cancer in CD-1 mice. *Oncogene* 23 (30) 5203-14

23. *Am J Physiol Endocrinol Metab* 2006 291(5):E906-12

24. Chobotova K, Vernallis AB, Majid FA (2010). Bromelain's

activity and potential as an anti-cancer agent: current evidence and perspectives. *Cancer Letter* 290 (2):148-56

25. Mehta R, Lansky EP (2004). Breast cancer chemopreventive properties of pomegranate (Punica Granatum) fruit extracts in a mouse mammary organ culture. *Eur J Cancer Prev* 13(4):345-8

26. Malik, A, et al (2005). Pomegranate fruit juice for chemoprevention and chemotherapy of prostate cancer. *Proceedings of the National Academy of Sciences*

27. Esmaillzadeh A et al (2006). Cholesterol-lowering effect of concentrated pomegranate juice consumption in Type II diabetic patients with hyperlipidemia. *Int J Vitam Nutr Res*; 76(3):147-51

28. Hartman, Richard E et al. Pomegranate juice decreases amyloid load and improves behaviour in a mouse model of Alzheimer's Disease. *Neurobiology of Disease* 24(3): 506-515

29. Ahmed, S et al. 2005. Punica Granatum L. Extract Inhibits IL-1beta-Induced Expression of Matrix Metalloproteinases by Inhibiting the Activation of MAP Kinases and NF KappaB in Human Chondrocytes in Vitro. *Journal of Nutrition* 135: 2096-2102

30. Menezes, Silvana MS, Cordeiro Luciano Nunes, Viana Glauce SB (2006). Punica granatum (Pomegranate) Extract is Active Against Dental Plaque. *Journal of Herbal Pharmacotherapy*, 6(2):79-92

Vegetables Week

1. Hung, HC; Joshipura, KJ; Jiang R, et al (2004). Fruit and vegetable intake and risk of major chronic disease. *J Natl Cancer Inst*. 96:1577-84

2. Boccardi, Virginia et al (2013). Mediterranean Diet, Telomere Maintenance and Health Status among Elderly. *PLOS* 8(4)

3. J. Webb et al (2008). Acute Blood Pressure Lowering,

Vasoprotective, and Antiplatelet Properties of Dietary Nitrate via Bioconversion to Nitrite. *Hypertension*, 2008; 51 (3)

4. Verhoeven DT et al (1997). A review of mechanisms underlying anticarcinogenicity by brassica vegetables. *Chem Biol Interact.* 103(2):79-129. (PubMed)

5. Conaway CC, Yang YM, Chung FL (2002). Isothiocyanates as cancer chemopreventive agents: their biological activities and metabolism in rodents and humans. *Curr Drug Metab.* 3(3):233-255. (PubMed)

6. Fahey JW, Zhang Y, Talalay P (1997). Broccoli sprouts: an exceptionally rich source of inducers of enzymes that protect against chemical carcinogens. *Proc Natl Acad Sci USA.* 94(19):10367-10372. (PubMed)

7. Kahlon TS, Chiu MC, Chapman MH (2008). Steam cooking significantly improves in vitro bile acid binding of collard greens, kale, mustard greens, broccoli, green bell pepper and cabbage. *Nutr Res* 28(6): 351-7

8. Zhang, W et al (2010). Allicin induces apoptosis in cancer cells through activation of both extrinsic and intrinsic pathways. *Oncol Rep* 24(6):1585-92

9. Fleischauer AT, Poole C, Arab L. (2000). Garlic consumption and cancer prevention: meta-analyses of colorectal and stomach cancers. *Am J Clin Nutr* 72(4):1047-1052

10. Kodama N et al (2002). Effects of D-fraction, a polysaccharide from Grifola frondosa on Tumor Growth Involve Activation of NK Cells. *Biological & Pharmaceutical Bulletin* 25, no. 12: 1647-1650

11. Edwards RF et al (2007). Quercetin reduces blood pressure in hypertensive subjects. *American Journal of Nutrition*

12. Jae-Hoon Jeong et al (2009). Effects of low-dose quercetin: cancer cell-specific inhibition of cell-cycle progression. *Journal of Cellular Biochemistry* 106(1) 73-82.)

13. You, W.C. et al (1989). Allium Vegetables and Reduced

Risk of Stomach Cancer. *Journal of the National Cancer Institute* 81, no. 2 162-164

14. Van Fenwyk J; Davis FG, Bowne, PE (1991). Dietary and serum carotenoids and cervical intraepithelial neoplasia. *International Journal of Cancer* 48:34-38

15. Giovannucci E et al (1995). Intake of carotenoids and retinol in relation to risk of prostate cancer. Journal of the *National Cancer Institute* 87(23):1767-1776

16. Sesso, H, et al (2003). Dietary lycopene, tomato-based food products, and cardiovascular disease in women. *Journal of Nutrition* 133(7):2336-41

Proteins Week

1. Pan et al (2012). Red meat consumption and mortality: Results from 2 Prospective Cohort Studies. *Archives of Internal Medicine* 0:201122871-9

2. Li D et al (2005). Lean meat and heart health. *Asia Pacific Journal of Clinical Nutrition* 14(2):113-9

3. Gorelik, Shlomit et al (2013). A rational approach to prevent postprandial modification of LDL by dietary polyphenols. *Journal of Functional Foods* 5(1):163-169

4. Micha Renata, RD, PhD; Wallace, Sarah K; Mozaffarian, Dariush MD (2010). Red and Processed Meat Consumption and Risk of Incident Coronary Heart Disease, Stroke, and Diabetes Mellitus. *Circulation*, 121:2271-2283

5. The World Cancer Research Fund/American Institute for Cancer Research. Food, Nutrition, Physical Activity, and the Prevention of Cancer: A Global Perspective. Washington, DC: AICR; 2007

6. Pan et al (2012). Red meat consumption and mortality: Results from 2 Prospective Cohort Studies. *Archives of Internal Medicine* 0:201122871-9

7. Sinha, Rashmi et al (2009). Meat Intake and Mortality – A Prospective Study of Over Half a Million People.

Archives of Internal Medicine 169(6):562-571

8. Peyaev M, Bashmakov Y K (2012). Could cheese be the missing piece of the French Paradox puzzle? *Medical Hypotheses* 79(6):746-9

9. Michaelsson, Karl et al (2014). Milk intake and risk of mortality and fractures in women and men: cohort studies. *BMJ* 27.10.2014

10. Levine, Morgan E et al (2014). Low Protein Intake Is Associated with a Major Reduction in IGF-1, Cancer, and Overall Mortality in the 65 and Younger but Not Older Population. *Cell Metabolism*, 2014; 19 (3): 407-417

11. Weinsier, Roland L; and Krumdieck, Carlos L (2000). Dairy foods and bone health: examination of the evidence1,2 *American Journal of Clinical Nutrition*, Vol. 72, No. 3, 681-689

12. Feskanich D et al (1997). Milk, dietary calcium, and bone fractures in women: a 12-year prospective study. *Am J Publ Health*;87:992-7

13. Vatanparast, Hassanali et al (2005). Positive effects of vegetable and fruit consumption and calcium intake on bone mineral accrual in boys during growth from childhood to adolescence: the University of Saskatchewan Pediatric Bone Mineral Accrual Study. *Am J Clin Nutr* 82(3):700-706

14. Mozaffarian, Dariush; Rimm, Eric. (2006). Fish intake, contaminants, and human health. *Journal of the American Medical Association*: 306(13); 1407-1501

15. Miller, Daphne, MD (2008). The Jungle Effect (William Morrow)

16. Mozaffarian, Dariush; Rimm, Eric. (2006). Fish intake, contaminants, and human health. *Journal of the American Medical Association*: 306(13); 1407-1501

17. Hu FB, Stampfer MJ, Rimm EB et al (1999). A prospective study of egg consumption and risk of cardiovascular disease in men and women. *JAMA* 281:1387-94

18. Tantamango YM et al (2011). Foods and food groups associated with the incidence of colorectal polyps: the Adventist Health Study. *Nutrition and Cancer* 63(4): 565-72

19. Trock B, Hilakivi-Clarke L, Clarke R(2006). Meta-Analysis of Soy Intake and Breast Cancer Risk. *Journal of the National Cancer Institute* 98:459-71

20. Peeters PH et al (2003). Phytoestrogens and breast cancer risk. Review of the epidemiological evidence. *Breast Cancer Res Treat*: 77(2):171-183

21. Helferich, WG et al (2004). Soy processing influences growth of estrogen-dependent breast cancer tumors. *Carcinogenesis*, 25 (9): 1649-57

22. Fraser Gary E (1999). Associations between diet and cancer, ischemic heart disease, and all-cause mortality in non-Hispanic white California Seventh Day Adventists . *American Journal of Clinical Nutrition*, 70(3): 532S-538S

Carbohydrates Week

1. Masters, Rachel C, et al (2010). Whole and Refined Grain Intakes are Related to Inflammatory Protein Concentrations in Human Plasma. *The Journal of Nutrition* 140(3):587-594

2. Tighe P, Duthie G, Vaughan N et al (2010). Effect of increased consumption of whole-grain foods on blood pressure and other cardiovascular risk markers in healthy middle-aged persons: a randomised controlled trial. *American Journal of Clinical Nutrition*. 92:733-740

3. Erkkila AT et al (2005). Cereal fiber and whole-grain intake are associated with reduced progression of coronary-artery atherosclerosis in postmenopausal women with coronary-artery disease. *American Heart Journal* 150(1): 94-101

4. Ling WH et al (2001). Red and Black Rice Decrease Levels of Atherosclerotic Plaque Formation and Increase Antioxidant Status in Rabbits. *Journal of Nutrition*

131(5):1421-6

5. Dewanto, V; Wu, Xiangzhong, Liu, Rui Hai, (2002). Processed sweet corn has higher antioxidant activity. *Journal of Agriculture and Food Chemistry* 50(17);4959-4964

6. *Ibid.*

Fats Week

1. Begin, M.E. et al (2004). Selective killing of human cancer cells by polyunsaturated fatty acids. *Prostaglandins, leukotrienes and medicine*. 19(2)177-186

2. Patterson, R.E., et al (2010). Marine Fatty Acid Intake is Associated with Breast Cancer Prognosis. *The Journal of Nutrition* 141(2):201-206

3. Appel LJ, Sacks FM, Carey VJ, et al (2005). Effects of protein, monounsaturated fats and carbohydrate intake on blood pressure and serum lipids: results of the Omniheart randomised trial. *JAMA* 294: 2455-64

4. Lahey, Richard et al (2014). Dietary Fat Supply to Failing Hearts Determines Dynamic Lipid Signaling for Nuclear Receptor Activation and Oxidation of Stored Triglyceride. *Circulation*, September 2014

5. Boyd, NF et al (2003). Dietetic guidelines on food and nutrition in the secondary prevention of cardiovascular disease – evidence from systematic reviews of randomised controlled trials. *Journal of Human Nutrition and Dietetics*. 19(6):401-419

6. Boyd NF et al (2003). Dietary fat and breast cancer risk revisited: a meta-analysis of the published literature. *British Journal of Cancer* 89(9): 1672-1685

7. Uchida, Koji (2007). Lipid peroxidation and redox-sensitive signalling pathways. *Current Atherosclerosis Reports* 9(3):216-221

8. Mozaffaria, D et al (2006). Trans- fatty acids and cardiovascular disease. *New England Journal of Medicine*. 354:1601-13

9. Tilakavati Karupaiah (1) and Kalyana Sundram (2). Effects of stereospecific positioning of fatty acids in triacylglycerol structures in native and randomized fats: a review of their nutritional implications. 1 Department of Nutrition & Dietetics, Faculty of Allied Health Sciences, National University of Malaysia, Jalan Raja Muda Abdul Aziz, Kuala Lumpur 50300, Malaysia. 2 Malaysian Palm Oil Council (MPOC), 2nd Floor Wisma Sawit, Lot 6, SS6 Jalan Perbandaran, 47301 Kelana Jaya, Selangor, Malaysia

Digestion Week

1. From http://en.wikipedia.org/wiki/List_of_countries_by_food_energy_intake
2. Chaix, Amandine et al (2014). Time-Restricted Feeding is a Preventative and Therapeutic Intervention Against Diverse Nutritional Challenges. *Cell Metabolism* 20(6):991-1005. Longo, Valter D; Fontana, Luigi (2010). Calorie restriction and cancer prevention: metabolic and molecular mechanisms. *Trends Pharmacol Sci*. 31(2):89-98
3. Lee C et al (2012). Fasting cycles retard growth of tumors and sensitize a range of cancer cell types to chemotherapy. *Sci Transl Med* 2012 Feb 8
4. Zhang Chenhong et al (2013). Structural modulation of gut microbiota in life-long calorie-restricted mice. *Nature Communications* article no: 2163

Probiotics Week

1. From Biocare. The Science of Probiotics at: file:///C:/Users/owner/Downloads/244-the-science-of-probiotics.pdf
2. Beare, Sally (2005). 50 Secrets of the World's Longest-Living People. (Avalon, USA)

Drinks Week

1. Ahmad N. et al (1997). Green Tea Constituent Epigallocatechin-3-gallate and Induction of Apoptosis and Cell Cycle Arrest in Human Carcinoma Cells. *Journal of the National Cancer Institute* 89(24): 1881-1886
2. Goto, K., Kanaya, S., and Hara, Y., (1991). Proceedings of the International Symposium on Tea Science (Shizuoka, Japan: The Organising Committee of ISTS), 314
3. Henning, SM et al (2012). Polyphenols in brewed green tea inhibit prostate cancer xenograft growth by localising to the tumor and decreasing oxidative stress and angiogenesis. *J Nutr Biochem* 23(11) 1537-42
4. Gorelik, Schlomit et al (2013). A rational approach to prevent postprandial modification of LDL by dietary polyphenols. *Journal of Functional Foods*, 5(1):163-169
5. Van Ginkel, Paul R (2007). Resveratrol Inhibits Tumor Growth of Human Neuroblastoma and Mediates Apoptosis by Directly Targeting Mitochondria. *Clinical Cancer Research* 13(5162)
6. Zoechlin, A., Liebner, F., Jungbauer, A. (2010). Red wine: a source of potent ligands for peroxisome proliferator-activated receptor gamma. *Food and Function* 10.1039/c0fo00086h
7. Parkin, D.M. (2011). Cancers attributable to consumption of alcohol in the UK in 2010. *British Journal of Cancer* 105; S14-S18

Week Ten

1. Dufault, R et al (2012). A macroepigenetic approach to identify factors responsible for the autism epidemic in the United States. *Clinical Epigenetics* 4:6
2. Joossens J.V. et al (1996). Dietary Salt, Nitrate and Stomach Cancer Mortality in 24 Countries. *International Journal of Epidemiology*. 25(3)494-502
3. Zhang, Z et al (2011). Habitual Coffee Consumption and

Risk of Hypertension: a Systematic Review and Meta-analysis of Prospective Observational Studies. *American Journal of Clinical Nutrition.* Keijzers, G.B. et al (2002). Caffeine Can Decrease Insulin Sensitivity in Humans. *Diabetes Care*

4. DE Koning, Lawrence et al (2012). Sweetened Beverage Consumption, Incidence Coronary Heart Disease, and Biomarkers of Risk in Men. *Circulation AHA* 111.067017

The Stacking Plan – what to do

Keep moving

1. Lee, IM (2012). Effect of physical inactivity on major non-communicable diseases worldwide: an analysis of burden of disease and life expectancy. *The Lancet* 380(9838): 219-229
2. Nicklett Emily J et al (2012). Fruit and Vegetable Intake, Physical Activity, and Mortality in Older Community-Dwelling Women. *Journal of the American Geriatrics Society* 60:862-868
3. Timothy S. Church et al MD, MPH, PhD et al (2007). Effects of Different Doses of Physical Activity on Cardiorespiratory Fitness Among Sedentary, Overweight or Obese Postmenopausal Women With Elevated Blood Pressure: A Randomized Controlled Trial *Journal of the American Medical Association* 2007;297:2081-2091
4. Simon B et al (2014). Extremely short duration high-intensity training substantially improves the physical function and self-reported health status of elderly adults *Journal of the American Geriatrics Society* 62(7):1380-1381
5. Merkel, Dr Drorit et al (2009), Chaim Sheba Medical Centre, Tel-Hashomer, *Journal of Adolescent Health* Sept 2009
6. The Third National Health and Nutrition Examination Survey 1994. Sunlight, Vitamin D, and Health. A

report of a conference held at the House of Commons in November 2005, organised by the Health Research Forum, UK

7. *Ibid.*
8. Dixon KM et al (2008). Skin cancer prevention: a possible role of 1,25dihydroxyvitamin D3 and its analogs. *J Steroid Biochem Mol Biol* 97(1-2):137-43
9. Viros A, Sanchez-Laorden B, Pedersen M, et al (2014). Ultraviolet radiation accelerates BRAF-driven melanomagenesis by targeting TP53. *Nature.* Published online June 11 2014

Relax

1. Sheldon Cohen (2007). Psychological Stress and Disease. *JAMA*, 298(14): 1685-7
2. Perls, T.T. and Silver, M.H., Living to 100, Basic Books, USA, 1999
3. Fekete, Erin M; Antoni, Michael H; Neil, Schneiderman (2007). 'Psychosocial and behavioural interventions for chronic medical conditions.' *Current Opinion in Psychiatry* 20 (2):152-157
4. Orme-Johnson, D.W. (1987). Medical Care Utilisation and the Transcendental Meditation Program. *Psychosomatic Medicine* 49:493-507
5. Moller-Levet, Carla S et al (2013). Effects of insufficient sleep on circadian rhythmicity and expression amplitude of the human blood transcriptome. *PNAS* 23.1.2013
6. Raikkonen K et al (2004). Sweet babies: chocolate consumption during pregnancy and infant temperament at six months. *Early Human Development* 76(2): 139-45
7. Lennox, S.S; Bedell, F.R., Stone A.A; (1990). 'The Effect of Exercise on Normal Mood', *Journal of Psychosomatic Research* 34, no 6:629-636

Make the connections

1. Office of National Statistics. Families and Households 2013/America's Families and Living Arrangements 2012, United States Census Bureau
2. The Way We Are Now: the state of the UK's relationships 2014. By Chris Sherwood, Dr Dylan Kneale and Barbara Bloomfield for Relate and Relationships Scotland
3. The Lonely Society? By Jo Griffin. The Mental Health Foundation, 2010
4. Loneliness amongst older people and the impact of family connections. WRVS, 2012
5. *www.telegraph.co.uk* 11th September 2013
6. House JS, Landis KR, Umberson D (1988). Social relationships and health. *Science* 241(4865):540-545
7. Holt-Lunstad, Julianne; Smith, Timothy B; Layton, J Bradley (2010). Social Relationships and Mortality Risk: A Meta-Analytic Review. *PLOS Medicine*, July 27
8. Giles, Lynne et al (2005). Effect of social networks on ten year survival in very old Australians: the Australian longitudinal study of aging. *Journal of Epidemiology and Community Health* 59; 574-579
9. Poulin, Michael et al (2013). Giving to Others and the Association between Stress and Mortality. *Am J Public Health*
10. Brown Stephen et al (2003). Providing Social Support May Be More Beneficial Than Receiving It. *Psychological Science* 14(4):320-7
11. Andrew Oswald and Jonathan Gardner (2002). 'Is it Money or Marriage that Keeps People Alive?'
12. Light, K.C., Grewen, K. M. and Amico, J.A.(2005). More Frequent Partner Hugs and Higher Oxytocin Levels Are Linked to Lower Blood Pressure and Heart Rate in Premenopausal Women. *Biological Psychology* 69 (1); 5-21
13. Kiekolt-Glaser J. K. et al (2005). Stress and wound healing *Arch Gen Psychiatry* 62:1377-1384

14. Zhang Hai et al (2013). Treatment of Obesity and Diabetes Using Oxytocin or Analogs in Patients and Mouse Models. *PLOS* 8(5)
15. Nagasawa, Miho, and Kikusui, Takefumi (2008). Pet dogs rival humans for emotional satisfaction. *Hormones and behaviour*

Have purpose

1. Boyle, Dr Patricia A et al (2009). Purpose in Life is Associated with Mortality Among Community-Dwelling Older Persons. *Psychosom Med* 71(5):574-579
2. Hill, Patrick; Turiano, Nicholas (2014). Purpose in life as a predictor of mortality across adulthood. *Psychological Science* 8 May 2014
3. Burrow, A. L., & HILL, P. L. (2013). Derailed by diversity?: Purpose buffers the relationship between ethnic composition on trains and passenger negative mood. *Personality and Social Psychology Bulletin, 39*, 1610-1619
4. Kim, Eric et al (2014). A Prospective Study of the Association Between Dispositional Optimism and Incident Heart Failure. *Circulation: Heart Failure*
5. Boyle, Dr Patricia A et al (2012). Effect of Purpose in Life on the Relation Between Alzheimer Disease Pathologic Changes on Cognitive Function in Advanced Age. *Archives of General Psychiatry* 69(5): 499-505
6. Tsai, Shan P et al (2005). Age at retirement and long term survival of an industrial population: prospective cohort study. *BMJ* 331(7523):995
7. Jacobs Tonya et al (2010). Intensive meditation training, immune cell telomerase activity, and psychological mediators. *Psychoneuroendocrinology*, 17th September 2010
8. From an article by James Hamblin entitled Health Tip: Find Purpose in Life published in *The Atlantic*, Nov 3rd 2014

Acknowledgements

I would like to thank my agent Sonia Land at Sheil Land Associates Ltd, William King at Akea for facilitating the writing of this book, Rebecca du Plessis at the Health Hub in Bristol for providing a fantastic venue in which to run *Stacking Plan* courses, Kris and Fran at Hub Radio for airing *Plate Date*, Jason Ewing at Group of Seven for the beautiful jacket design, Ollie and Claire for being wonderful 'human guinea pigs', and Simon for a range of technical, electronic and pastoral support.

About the Author

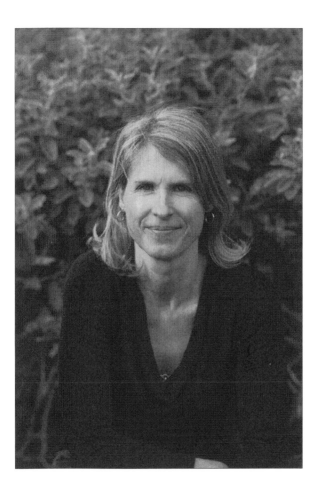

Sally Beare, dip BCNH, CNHC, is a nutritional therapist and author who trained at the UK College of Nutrition and Health in London (BCNH). She lives and works in Bristol where she sees clients, runs healthy-eating programmes and gives nutrition workshops in schools. She has also lectured on anti-ageing at BCNH. Sally has travelled all over the world in her quest to discover the eating and living habits of ultra-healthy, long lived populations.

Sally is the author of *50 Secrets of the World's Longest-Living People* (Avalon, US, 2006) and *The Live-Longer Diet*, (Piatkus, UK, 2003). Her books have been widely acclaimed and translated into many different languages worldwide. *The Stacking Plan* is her third book.

Printed in Great Britain
by Amazon